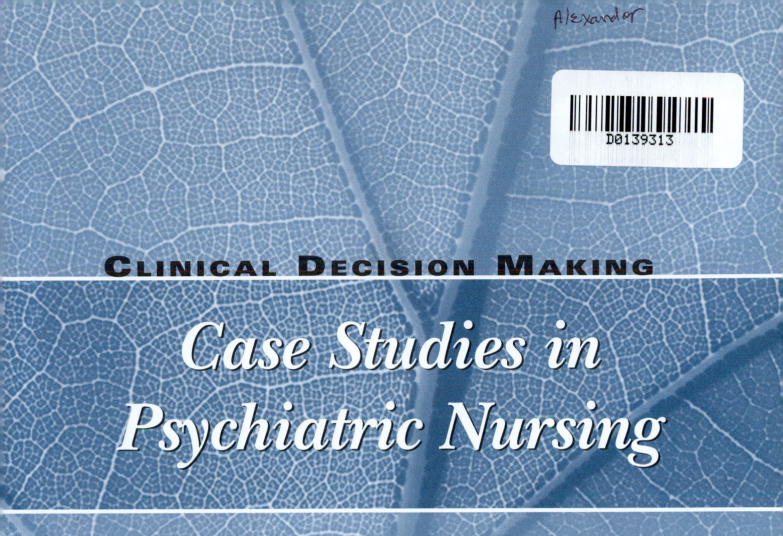

CLINICAL DECISION MAKING

Case Studies in Psychiatric Nursing

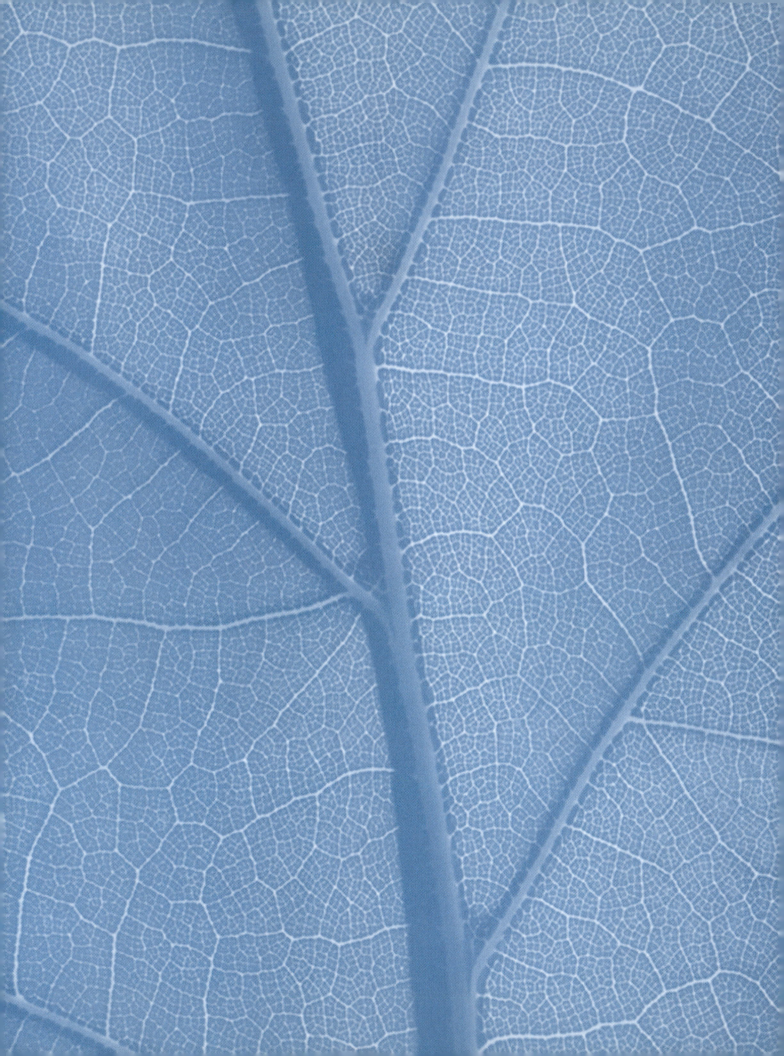

CLINICAL DECISION MAKING

Case Studies in Psychiatric Nursing

Betty Kehl Richardson

PhD, RN, CNS-MHP, BC, LPC, LMFT

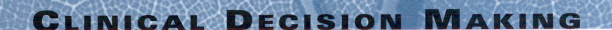

THOMSON

DELMAR LEARNING

Australia   Canada   Mexico   Singapore   Spain   United Kingdom   United States

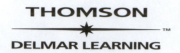

THOMSON
DELMAR LEARNING

Clinical Decision Making: Case Studies in Psychiatric Nursing
by Betty Kehl Richardson, PhD, RN, CNS-MHP, BC, LPC, LMFT

**Vice President,
Health Care Business Unit:**
William Brottmiller

Director of Learning Solutions:
Matthew Kane

Acquisitions Editor:
Maureen Rosener

Product Manager:
Elizabeth Howe

Editorial Assistant:
Chelsey Iaquinta

Marketing Director:
Jennifer McAvey

Marketing Manager:
Michele McTighe

Marketing Coordinator:
Danielle Pacella

Production Director:
Carolyn Miller

Content Project Manager:
Jessica McNavich

Library of Congress Cataloging-in-Publication Data

Richardson, Betty Kehl.
   Clinical decision making: case studies in psychiatric nursing / Betty Kehl Richardson.
      p. ; cm.
   Includes bibliographical references and index.
   ISBN 1-4018-3845-6 (pbk. : alk. paper)
   1. Psychiatric nursing—Case studies. 2. Nursing assessment—Case studies. I. Title.
   [DNLM: 1. Psychiatric Nursing—Case Reports. WY 160 R521c 2007]
   RC440.R53 2007
   616.89'0231—dc22

                                          2006015980

Notice to the Reader

Contents

Reviewers

Ann K. Beckett, PhD, RN
Assistant Professor
Oregon Health and Science University School of Nursing
Portland, Oregon

Jane E. Bostick, PhD, APRN, BC
Assistant Professor of Clinical Nursing
University of Missouri–Columbia
Sinclair School of Nursing
Columbia, Missouri

Kimberly M. Gregg, MS APRN, BC
Adult Mental Health Clinical Nurse Specialist
Altru Health Systems
Instructor
University of North Dakota
Grand Forks, North Dakota

Bethany Phoenix, RN, PhD, CNS
Associate Clinical Professor
Coordinator, Graduate Program in Psychiatric/Mental Health Nursing
University of California, San Francisco
San Francisco, California

Charlotte R. Price, EdD, RN
Professor and Chair
Augusta State University Department of Nursing
Augusta, Georgia

Linda Stafford, PhD, RN, CS
Division Head, Psychiatric Mental Health Nursing
The University of Texas Health Science Center at Houston
School of Nursing
Houston, Texas

Preface

Thomson Delmar Learning's Case Studies Series was created to encourage nurses to bridge the gap between content knowledge and clinical application. The products within the series represent the most innovative and comprehensive approach to nursing case studies ever developed. Each title has been authored by experienced nurse educators and clinicians who understand the complexity of nursing practice as well as the challenges of teaching and learning. All of the cases are based on real-life clinical scenarios and demand thought and "action" from the nurse. Each case brings the user into the clinical setting, and invites him or her to utilize the nursing process while considering all of the variables that influence the client's condition and the care to be provided. Each case also represents a unique set of variables, to offer a breadth of learning experiences and to capture the reality of nursing practice. To gauge the progression of a user's knowledge and critical thinking ability, the cases have been categorized by difficulty level. Every section begins with basic cases and proceeds to more advanced scenarios, thereby presenting opportunities for learning and practice for both students and professionals.

All of the cases have been expert reviewed to ensure that as many variables as possible are represented in a truly realistic manner and that each case reflects consistency with realities of modern nursing practice.

Praise for Delmar Learning's Case Study Series

"These cases show diversity and richness of content and should stimulate lively discussions with students."

—LINDA STAFFORD, PhD, RN
Division Head, Psychiatric Mental Health
Nursing, School of Nursing, The University of
Texas Health Science Center at Houston

"The use of case studies is pedagogically sound and very appealing to students and instructors. I think that some instructors avoid them because of the challenge of case development. You have provided the material for them."

—NANCY L. OLDENBURG, RN, MS, CPNP
Clinical Instructor, Northern Illinois University

"[The author] has done an excellent job of assisting students to engage in critical thinking. I am very impressed with the cases, questions, and content. I rarely ask that students buy more than one . . . book . . . but, in this instance, I can't wait until this book is published."

—DEBORAH J. PERSELL, MSN, RN, CPNP
Assistant Professor, Arkansas State University

"[The case studies] are very current and prepare students for the twenty-first-century mental health arena."

—CHARLOTTE R. PRICE, EdD, RN
Professor and Chair, Augusta State University
Department of Nursing

"One thing I always tell my students is that they will encounter mental health issues in all the various areas of nursing that they practice. Often they don't grasp this concept. . . . Many mental health nursing books focus on mental health settings and miss the other settings. I appreciate the fact that different settings were used in this reading . . . inpatient and outpatient, as well as med-surg, plastic surgery, etc."

—KIMBERLY M. GREGG, MS APRN, BC
Adult Mental Health Clinical Nurse Specialist,
Altru Health Systems, Instructor, University of
North Dakota

"This is a groundbreaking book. . . . This book should be a required text for all undergraduate and graduate nursing programs and should be well-received by faculty."

—JANE H. BARNSTEINER, PhD, RN, FAAN
Professor of Pediatric Nursing, University of
Pennsylvania School of Nursing

How to Use this Book

Every case begins with a table of variables that are encountered in practice, and that must be understood by the nurse in order to provide appropriate care to the client. Categories of variables include age, gender, setting, ethnicity, cultural considerations, preexisting conditions, coexisting conditions, communication considerations, disability considerations, socioeconomic considerations, spiritual considerations, pharmacological considerations, psychosocial considerations, legal considerations, ethical considerations, alternative therapy, prioritization considerations, and delegation considerations. If a case involves a variable that is considered to have a significant impact on care, the specific variable is included in the table. This allows the user an "at a glance" view of the issues that will need to be considered to provide care to the client in the scenario. The table of variables is followed by a presentation of the case, including the history of the client, current condition, clinical setting, and professionals involved. A series of questions follows each case that ask the user to consider how she would handle the issues presented within the scenario. Suggested answers and rationales are provided for remediation and discussion.

Organization

Cases are grouped according to psychiatric disorder. Within each part, cases are organized by difficulty level from easy, to moderate, to difficult. This classification is somewhat subjective, but they are based upon a developed standard. In general, difficulty level has been determined by the number of variables that impact the case and the complexity of the client's condition. Colored tabs are used to allow the user to distinguish the difficulty levels more easily. A comprehensive table of variables is also provided for reference, to allow the user to quickly select cases containing a particular variable of care.

The cases are fictitious; however, they are based on actual problems and/or situations the nurse will encounter. Any resemblance to actual cases or individuals is coincidental.

Acknowledgments

For the invitation to write this book, the author wishes to express her appreciation to Erin Silk and Matt Kane of Thomson Delmar Publishers. A number of product managers and staff were involved over time, and the author thanks them for their help. The author is most indebted to Elizabeth (Libby) Howe, the final product manager, who provided guidance, feedback, ideas, and encouragement to keep the project alive and get the book into print. Another special thanks goes to Nora Armbruster, who managed the final production stage and made it possible to meet the print deadline. The author wants to especially thank the reviewers and copy editors of this book, for their time, expertise, critical comments, and suggestions, which resulted in changes to make the book much better.

A number of colleagues at Austin Community College, Austin, Texas; Austin State Hospital; and Seton Shoal Creek Psychiatric Hospital, as well as other psychiatric and medical facilities, were consulted about selected aspects of the cases to verify accuracy and currency. The author recognizes and appreciates the important contributions of these colleagues: Sally Samford, Marita Peppard, Donna Edwards, Kris Benton, Kitty Viek, Jane Luetchens, and many others.

Teachers and school nurses were consulted, as were parents of children with special issues. The author wishes to recognize their important contributions, especially Edna Nation, who teaches high school students in Liberty Hill, Texas, for her dedication to helping all students—including those with medical and mental health problems—achieve their maximum potential and for sharing her ideas with the author.

The author thanks her family and friends for their patience and understanding during the long months of research and writing. This project could not have been finished without their encouragement and cooperation.

Dedication

This book is dedicated to my son Mark, who has battled cancer throughout most of the time this book was in progress. Sharing with me some of his innermost thoughts, fears, and struggles has reinforced for me that what student nurses, family, and others see on the surface in a brief interaction with a client can be a very different picture than what is going on inside the client. Compassion, empathy, and therapeutic communication do help us understand that inner person. I am indebted to Mark for all he has taught me.

Additionally, this book is dedicated to all the good nurses in various fields of nursing, not just psychiatric mental health nursing, who apply psychiatric techniques and principles when working with clients who have mental health diagnoses and/or issues.

Note from the Author

These case studies were designed to help nursing students at all levels to not only fine tune their critical thinking skills and their therapeutic communication skills, but to develop a deeper understanding of, and empathy for, clients who have what we currently refer to as psychiatric problems. The mind and body are inseparable, so physical health problems are interwoven with mental health problems within the cases. The student nurse, and anyone else who reads these case studies, is encouraged to ask themselves: "What is the most therapeutic approach or response to this client in this situation?" as they answer the questions within the cases.

About the Author

Dr. Richardson began a nursing career in 1959 as a new diploma graduate. She worked five years in obstetrical nursing at Memorial Medical Center, Springfield, Illinois; much of this time she worked in the labor rooms and applied nearly everything she learned in psychiatric nursing to emotionally support laboring women, new mothers, and grieving parents who lost babies. She next worked as an office nurse for Dr. Tom Masters, a general internist who specialized in Diabetes. The following several years she worked for the Illinois Department of Mental Health Mental Retardation, working on an outpatient team serving three rural counties. The team followed the blurred role concept in which every member did intake evaluations and did counseling with people having the full range of diagnoses and issues possible in mental health work. This work stimulated a return to school for a bachelor's in nursing and a master's in administration from the University of Illinois at Springfield, a master's degrees in adult nursing from the Medical College of Georgia, and a PhD in psychiatric mental health nursing from the University of Texas at Austin, Texas. Her dissertation was "The Psychiatric Inpatient's Perception of the Seclusion Room Experience." She published the results of this study in *Nursing Research*. Dr. Richardson has taught in an RN to BSN program, two ADN programs, and a licensed vocational nursing program. She received the NISOD teaching award for teaching excellence from the University of Texas.

Throughout the years, volunteer work has been a passion. Dr. Richardson made fifteen trips to Honduras and Nicaragua with MEDICO, a nonprofit organization taking medical, eye, and dental care to remote areas that are medically underserved. She co-led trips to the Moskito Coast of Nicaragua and Honduras and volunteered for several months in a program to take boys off the streets of LaCeiba, Honduras. Additional volunteer work has been with the homeless in Austin, Texas.

Dr. Richardson is also a licensed professional counselor and a licensed marriage and family therapist and has done therapy for over thirty years (full time and part time). She has worked as a therapist in a residential program for children and adolescents and as a service administrator and therapist on a child/adolescent unit in a private psychiatric hospital. She led weekend groups in a private psychiatric hospital for many years while teaching full time. She was Director of Nursing of Austin State Hospital, Austin, Texas, for six years. Over the years, Dr. Richardson has had training with a number of the great theorists such as Bettleheim, Azrin, Frankl, Ellis, and others. She has had training in a variety of therapies from Psychoanalytic Theory to Play Therapy to Brief Psychotherapy. She is a board-certified clinical specialist in child adolescent psychiatric nursing (certified by the American Nurses Association). She continues in her private practice, works part time in a drug study clinic, freelances for publishers, and has written a monthly column for parents in the newsmagazine *Austin Parent* since 1992. Dr. Richardson has lived in Austin, Texas, for over twenty-five years, and she can be contacted there by e-mail at bkrich@sbcglobal.net.

Comprehensive Table of Variables

Case Study	Gender	Age	Setting	Ethnicity	Culture	Preexisting Conditions	Coexisting Conditions	Communication	Disability	Socioeconomic Status	Spirituality	Pharmacologic	Psychosocial	Legal	Ethical	Alternative Therapy	Prioritization	Delegation
Part One: The Client Experiencing Schizophrenia and Other Psychotic Disorders																		
1	F	34	Psychiatric hospital	Hungarian American	X		X					X	X	X	X			
2	M	48	Clinic	American Indian/White American	X	X				X		X	X	X	X	X		
Part Two: The Client Experiencing Anxiety																		
1	M	26	Outpatient	White American			X					X	X	X				
2	F	50	Center	Mexican American	X					X		X	X		X	X		
3	F	19	Psychiatric hospital	White American	X						X	X	X					
4	F	25	Hospital	Central American	X		X					X	X	X	X			
Part Three: The Client Experiencing Depression or Mania																		
1	M	14	Psychiatric hospital	Black American	X		X			X	X	X	X	X	X		X	X
2	F	35	Inpatient psych. hosp.	Central American				X		X		X		X	X		X	X
3	F	13	Psychiatric hospital	White American	X		X			X	X		X		X	X	X	X
4	F	41	Hospital	German	X		X					X	X	X	X		X	X
Part Four: The Client Who Abuses Chemical Substances																		
1	M	42	Hospital	White American	X		X			X	X		X	X	X	X	X	X
2	F	51	Home	White American	X	X	X		X	X	X	X	X	X	X	X	X	
3	M	19	Office	White American	X					X			X	X	X			
4	F	13	School nurse	White American	X	X									X			X
Part Five: The Client with a Personality Disorder																		
1	F	27	Office	White American	X		X			X	X		X	X	X		X	X
2	M	39	Center	White American	X					X		X	X	X	X	X	X	
3	M	55	Home	White American	X	X				X	X		X	X	X	X	X	X
4	M	62	Clinic	White American	X	X	X			X	X		X	X	X	X		
5	F	22	Center	White American			X			X			X	X	X		X	X
6	M	36	ER	White American			X				X	X	X	X	X		X	
7	M	32	Clinic	Black/White American	X		X					X	X	X	X	X	X	X

Part Six: The Client Experiencing a Somatoform, Factitious, or Dissociative Disorder

	Sex	Age	Setting	Ethnicity
1	F	15	ER	White/Chilean American
2	F	51	Home	African American
3	F	34	Psychiatric unit	White American
4	F	31	Office	White American

Part Seven: The Client with Disorders of Self-Regulation

	Sex	Age	Setting	Ethnicity
1	F	26	Psychiatric hospital	White American
2	F	21	Hospital	East Asian/White American
3	M	25	Local jail	White American

Part Eight: Special Populations: The Child, Adolescent, or Elderly Client

	Sex	Age	Setting	Ethnicity
1	M	13	Center	White American
2	M	14	Hospital	White American
3	F	8	School nurse	White American
4	F	7	School nurse	Asian American
5	M	5	Children's unit	Asian American
6	F	7	School nurse	White American
7	F	89	Home	Black American
8	M	15	School	White/Black American
9	M	7	Center	White American

Part Nine: Survivors of Violence or Abuse

	Sex	Age	Setting	Ethnicity
1	F	10	Home	White American
2	M	77	Gerontologist's office	White American
3	M	11	School infirmary	White/Hispanic American

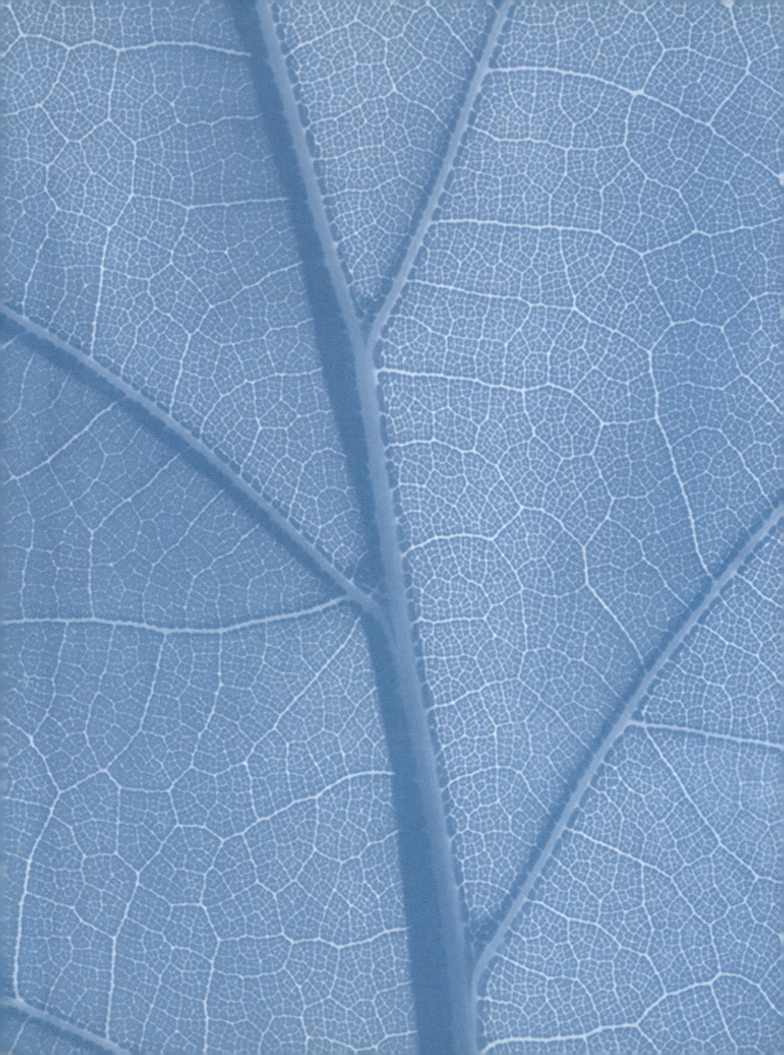

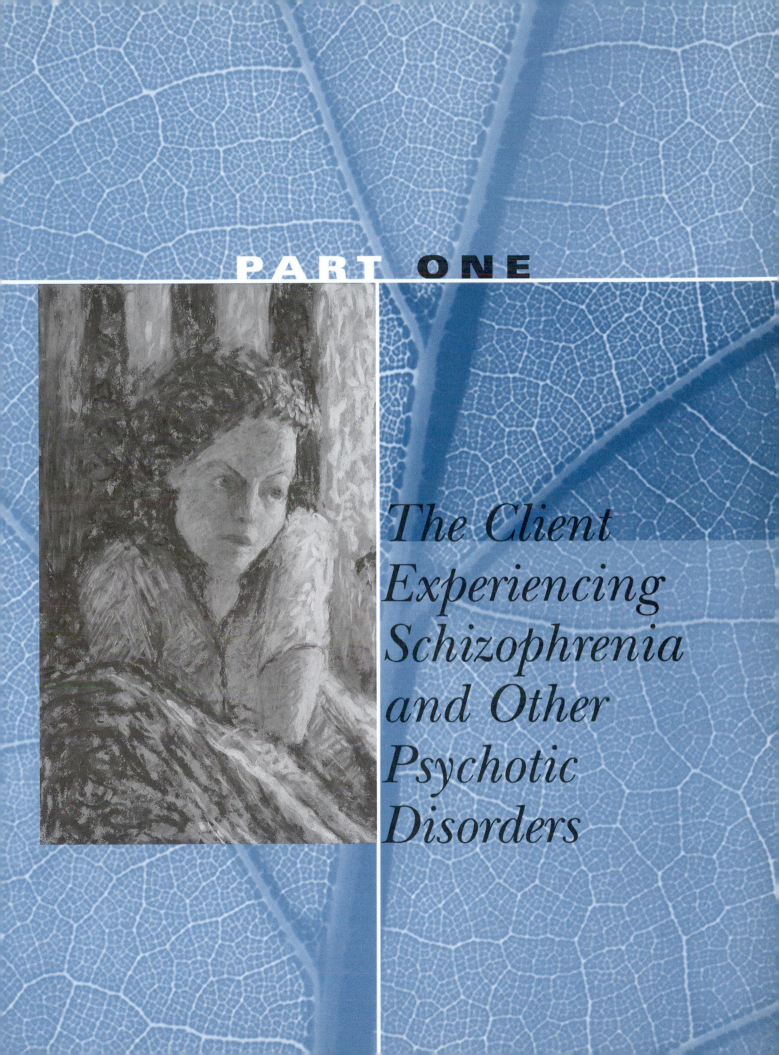

PART ONE

The Client Experiencing Schizophrenia and Other Psychotic Disorders

Sarah

GENDER

Female

AGE

34

SETTING

- Psychiatric hospital

ETHNICITY

- Hungarian American

CULTURAL CONSIDERATIONS

- Hungarian customs

PREEXISTING CONDITION

COEXISTING CONDITION

COMMUNICATION

DISABILITY

SOCIOECONOMIC

SPIRITUAL/RELIGIOUS

PHARMACOLOGIC

- Valproic acid (Depakote)
- Risperodone (Risperdal) liquid
- Venlafaxine hydrochloride (Effexor XR)

PSYCHOSOCIAL

LEGAL

- Confidentiality
- Consent
- Client's rights
- Release of information

ETHICAL

ALTERNATIVE THERAPY

PRIORITIZATION

DELEGATION

SCHIZOAFFECTIVE DISORDER, BIPOLAR TYPE

Level of difficulty: Moderate

Overview: Requires familiarity with the current diagnostic requirements for Schizoaffective Disorder and approaches to the psychotic client, including checking the client's mouth to prevent cheeking of medications. Requires critical thinking about accepting gifts from clients.

Client Profile

Sarah is a 34-year-old female. Born in Hungary, she married an American and came to this country when she was 25 years old. About a year later, Sarah began a series of admissions to psychiatric facilities. She was diagnosed with major depression and later with Schizoaffective Disorder. About a month ago, Sarah stopped keeping outpatient appointments, stopped taking her medication, stopped bathing, and stopped eating, but was sleeping all the time. Sarah's mood symptoms suddenly became less noticeable, and she began wandering her yard after dark, saying the neighbors were in the trees. Sarah began to carry a gun to protect herself against the neighbors, who she thought were out to kill her. When she started to fire the gun into the trees, her brother got a court order to have Sarah committed for treatment.

Case Study

Two deputies, one male and one female, and her brother have brought Sarah to the psychiatric hospital to be admitted. The nurse does an assessment on Sarah and discovers Sarah has been on risperodone (Risperdal) liquid, valproic acid (Depakote), and venlafaxine (Effexor XR). The psychiatrist orders these medications to be continued. At first the nurse is unable to get Sarah to sign consent forms to take the medication, but after a few days, she does sign the forms. By this time, her pregnancy test has come back negative, and she is started back on her usual medication.

The nurse finds Sarah to be somewhat tangential with loose associations. When the nurse assigns Sarah to attend a medication class, she refuses. When asked to interpret a proverb, she refuses.

Sarah begins to talk about her food being poisoned and being "king" of the hospital. She claims to have subjects to take care of the food and those who try to poison it.

Sarah tells the nurse that she has been hospitalized eight times previously at another psychiatric facility. The nurse sends a signed release of information form to the designated psychiatric facility requesting copies of Sarah's latest psychosocial assessment, treatment plan, and discharge summary. The requested information reveals that Sarah's discharge diagnosis at that facility was Schizoaffective Disorder, Bipolar Type.

After three weeks on medication, Sarah no longer seems to have hallucinations and delusions. The psychiatrist is ready to discharge Sarah, but her Depakote level comes back low. A nurse discovers Sarah has been cheeking her morning dose and sometimes her evening dose of Depakote and has been putting the medicine in a pair of shoes.

Sarah hands the nurse an envelope with two hundred dollars and the words "Thank-you nurse" written on the outside. About this time the nurse notices that Sarah has suddenly become hyperverbal, hyperactive, intrusive, and sexually suggestive to peers and staff.

Questions

1. What is Schizoaffective Disorder?

2. Do Sarah's symptoms match those of Schizoaffective Disorder, and if so, how?

3. On what basis do you think Sarah was court committed?

4. Why was Sarah's medication delayed? Why did the nurse not start it on admission?

5. Why does the nurse ask Sarah to interpret a proverb?

6. Does Sarah have hallucinations and/or delusions? What makes you think so?

7. What is the age of onset, the male to female ratio, and the prevalence of Schizoaffective Disorder?

8. Discuss the current theories of etiology, treatment, and prognosis of Schizoaffective Disorder.

9. What nursing diagnoses would you most likely write for Sarah?

10. What goals and interventions do you suggest for Sarah for one of these nursing diagnoses?

11. What are the possible explanations for the client giving the nurse an envelope with money in it? How would you respond to this gift offer if you were the nurse?

CASE STUDY 2

Dean

GENDER

Male

AGE

48

SETTING

- Community clinic for low-income clients

ETHNICITY

- American Indian and White American

CULTURAL CONSIDERATIONS

- Pima Indian culture

PREEXISTING CONDITION

- Diabetes

COEXISTING CONDITION

- Cough, fever

COMMUNICATION

DISABILITY

SOCIOECONOMIC

- Homeless

SPIRITUAL/RELIGIOUS

PHARMACOLOGIC

- Metformin (Glucophage)
- Risperodone (Risperdal)
- Trihexyphenidyl (Artane)
- Benztropine (Cogentin)

PSYCHOSOCIAL

- Isolating

LEGAL

- Confidentiality
- Consent for release of information

ETHICAL

- Respect for client's lifestyle choices (paternalism vs. autonomy)

ALTERNATIVE THERAPY

- Medicine man to overcome sources of evil influence on his life

PRIORITIZATION

DELEGATION

SCHIZOPHRENIA

Level of difficulty: Moderate

Overview: Requires the nurse to self-assess feelings about working with a homeless mentally ill client with diabetes and symptoms of Tardive Dyskinesia. The nurse must consider the client's Native American culture.

Client Profile

Dean, a 48 year-old male, grew up on a Pima Indian reservation in Arizona. He left the reservation after high school to serve in the army but was diagnosed and treated for Schizophrenia at age 21 and was discharged early. He has been in and out of psychiatric facilities for several years. He periodically takes a bus back to the reservation to see a medicine man, but he does not stay as he has no work and only distant, poor family there.

Case Study

Dean has come to the community health center. While he is sitting in the lobby, the nurse observes Dean without him being aware of this. The nurse notices that at times he seems to be talking to the air around him. She also notices that Dean is smacking his lips, his tongue protrudes at times, and he periodically coughs without covering his mouth.

When it is time for the nurse to do an assessment on Dean, the receptionist notifies the nurse that Dean has not filled out the intake form. The nurse tries to help him by asking him for his address. Although his speech is somewhat disorganized at times, the nurse finds out from Dean that he is homeless and currently living on the streets. His chief complaint is "not feeling well." The nurse takes Dean's vital signs, which are: T. 100.4, R. 22, P. 100, BP 152/98. He is 5 foot 8 inches tall and weighs 235 pounds. When weighed he says he has recently lost thirty pounds.

When the nurse asks Dean what medications he is on, he shows her some empty medicine bottles, saying he has run out of his medication and does not have the money to buy more. The labels on the bottles indicate he is on metformin (Glucophage), an oral antidiabetic medication, and risperodone (Risperdal). The nurse asks him why he takes Risperdal and also inquires about other medication he has taken in the past. He replies that he was diagnosed with Schizophrenia at age 21 and that he was on Thorazine for several years, then Haldol, then Prolixin injections, and maybe some he forgot before the current Risperdal. He explains that he has gone to the community mental health center twice to get more Risperdal samples

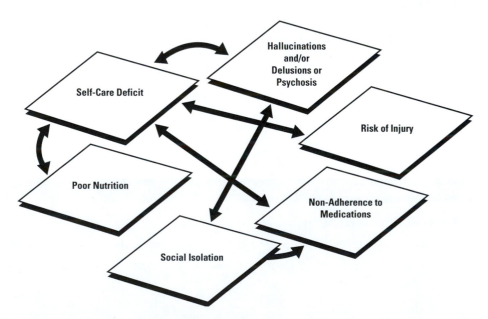

Concept map of issues and problems associated with schizophrenia

and waited most of the day each time without being seen by the psychiatrist. Dean says he either lost, or someone stole, his last supply of Risperdal, so he has not been taking it for about a month. The nurse suspects Dean is hearing voices.

When asked about any health problems, he says he has diabetes, which he is supposed to "keep under control with diet and pills." He also complains of a cough, something the nurse noticed earlier. After the nurse develops some rapport with Dean, he tells her about seeing and hearing an owl that frightens him. He talks about needing to see a medicine man.

Questions

1. What are some feelings that nurses could have about working with people who are homeless and mentally ill, and why would it be important for a nurse to think about his or her feelings toward this population?

2. Discuss the possible significance of Dean's appearance and observed behaviors.

3. What screening tests and/or lab procedures seem to be indicated?

4. What is Tardive Dyskinesia, how common is it, and what is the treatment for it? What did the nurse observe about Dean that would suggest Tardive Dyskinesia?

5. Is diabetes common among persons with a diagnosis of Schizophrenia? Is diabetes more common among Native American Indians? Discuss the possibility of persons with Schizophrenia having medical problems.

6. What precautions should the nurse take with the homeless population?

7. What additional information about Dean would be helpful, and how could this be obtained? What reason can you think of for Dean wanting to see a medicine man?

8. What findings by the health team would be sufficient to get Dean hospitalized in a psychiatric facility, and what opportunities might hospitalization present?

9. What findings might get this client hospitalized in a general hospital, and what opportunities might that present?

10. If you were the nurse in this case, would you want to get Dean off the street and into some other type of living situation? Why or why not? What reasons could he have for wanting to continue living on the streets?

11. Discuss resources likely to be available in the community for the homeless mentally ill, such as food, clothing, shelter, and medical care.

12. What nursing diagnoses and interventions would you write for this client?

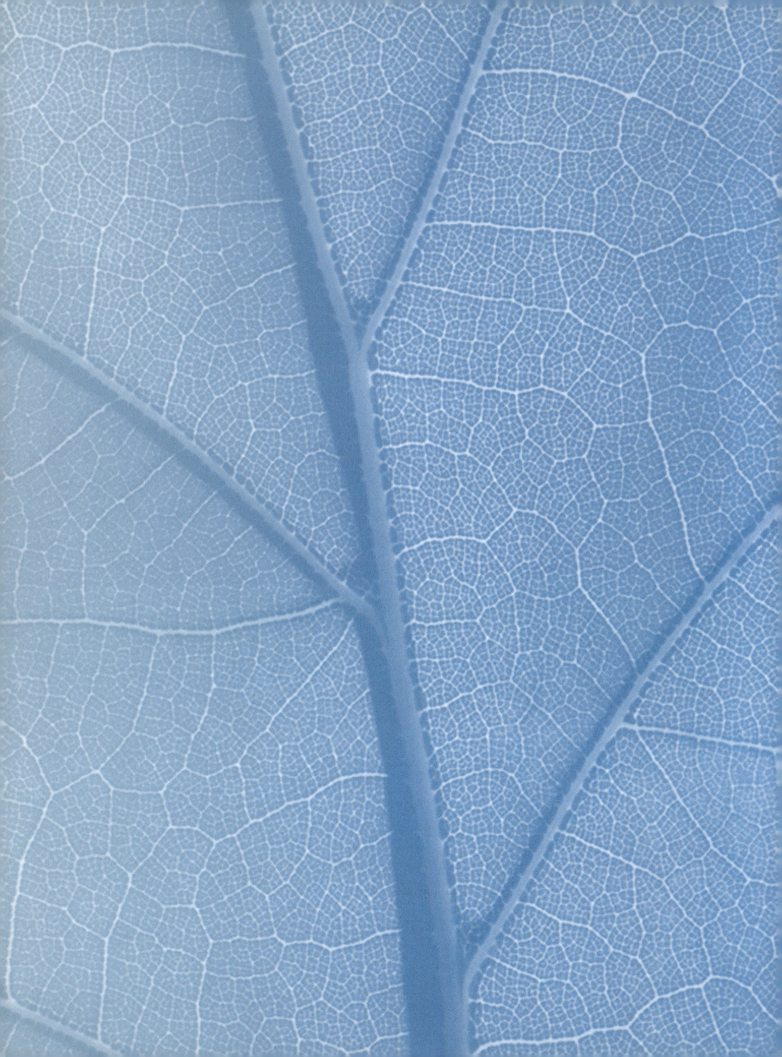

PART TWO

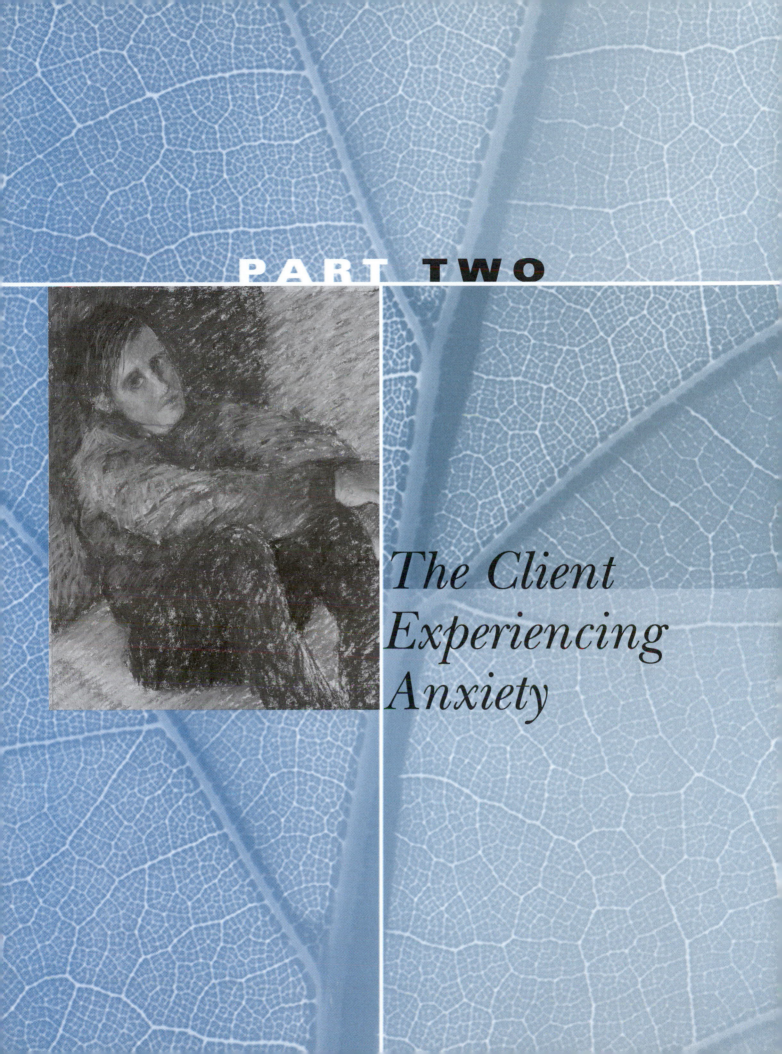

*The Client
Experiencing
Anxiety*

Jim

GENDER

Male

AGE

26

SETTING

- Evening outpatient treatment program

ETHNICITY

- White American

CULTURAL CONSIDERATIONS

PREEXISTING CONDITION

COEXISTING CONDITION

- Alcoholism

COMMUNICATION

DISABILITY

SOCIOECONOMIC

SPIRITUAL/RELIGIOUS

PHARMACOLOGIC

- Refusal to eat with or in front of others limits socialization
- Socialization revolves around alcohol

PSYCHOSOCIAL

LEGAL

- Confidentiality
- Informed consent
- DWI

ETHICAL

ALTERNATIVE THERAPY

PRIORITIZATION

DELEGATION

MODERATE

SOCIAL PHOBIA (SOCIAL ANXIETY DISORDER)

Level of difficulty: Moderate

Overview: Requires nurse to use therapeutic communication techniques. The nurse must also use critical thinking to identify her own thinking errors, teach the client and peers to recognize and correct thinking errors, and develop a care plan for a client with dual diagnosis: Social Phobia and Alcohol Abuse.

Client Profile

Jim is a 26-year-old husband and father of a preschool child. He lives and works in a small town in the finance department of an automobile dealership. The main places to gather socially in this small town are churches and bars. Jim prefers the bars where he can watch sports on T.V., talk to people, and drink "a couple of beers" with coworkers and friends. Jim's plan to drink a couple of beers usually turns into a dozen or more beers.

Jim never eats with anyone from work and usually turns down all social engagements that he and his wife are invited to. If he has to attend a work-related social event, he has a feeling that others are looking at him and judging him and he experiences tremors, palpitations, and sweating. Jim never accepts anything to eat at these events. Friends have stopped inviting Jim and his wife to dinner as the invitations are always declined. Jim tells his best friend: "I just don't feel comfortable eating in front of other people. I am afraid I will do something embarrassing and humiliate myself. This sounds unreasonable, even to me; but that is just the way that I am." Jim has been offered a job that pays more money and has better hours, but he would have to take clients to lunch and dinner. He has turned this job down due to his extreme discomfort with eating in public or with anyone other than his immediate family.

Case Study

Jim is attending a nightly outpatient chemical abuse treatment program as part of his follow-up after an inpatient program for substance abuse, a deal his lawyer worked out after he was found guilty of driving while intoxicated. The nurse at the treatment program notices that Jim does not go to the cafeteria with the rest of his group for the evening meal but sits alone in the lobby watching sports on television. The nurse wonders if Jim has enough money to buy dinner and begins to worry that he will be hungry when she does the medication education group later. She thinks about offering him half of her sandwich she brought from home, but stops herself from doing this as she recognizes she has committed a thinking error. The nurse has begun to wonder about Jim and why he seems so reticent, so hesitant to answer questions or share in group sessions or the community meetings. Last time

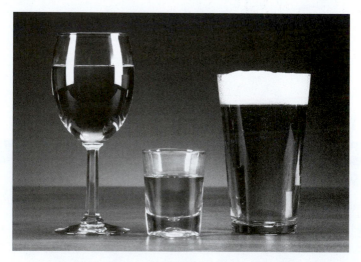

About 20% of clients with social anxiety disorder also have an alcohol use disorder.

she asked him a question in the community meeting, his face flushed and peers teased him, saying he was blushing like a girl and accusing him of having a crush on the nurse.

The nurse approaches Jim and says: "I notice you did not go to eat with your group."

Questions

1. Was the nurse's decision not to offer Jim half of her sandwich a good idea or not? Give a rationale for your answer. What else could the nurse do?

2. What do you think is the rationale for the nurse's opening remark: "I notice you did not go to eat with your group"? What therapeutic communication techniques are you familiar with that could be used in communication with Jim?

3. How do you think the nurse could best deal with the peers' comments about Jim blushing?

4. What is Social Phobia? Do you think this client has signs and symptoms that match those of Social Phobia (Social Anxiety Disorder)? Give a rationale for your answer.

5. Are there any differences in the signs and symptoms of children with Social Phobia compared to those of adults?

6. What are some theories of causation of Social Phobia?

7. What is the incidence of Social Phobia?

8. What other disorders or problems are common in the population experiencing Social Phobia? Could there be a connection between this client's drinking and Social Phobia (Social Anxiety Disorder)? If so, how would you assess for a connection?

9. What is the current thinking about heredity and alcohol abuse? What are some current treatments for those with early onset alcoholism?

10. What are some of the current treatments being used to treat Social Phobia?

11. What nursing diagnoses would you likely write for this client?

12. Discuss possible goals and interventions for this client. Is it possible to treat the alcoholism and the Social Phobia concurrently?

Betty

GENDER

Female

AGE

50

SETTING

- Community mental health center

ETHNICITY

- Mexican American

CULTURAL CONSIDERATIONS

- Hispanic

PREEXISTING CONDITION

COEXISTING CONDITION

COMMUNICATION

DISABILITY

SOCIOECONOMIC

- Daughter of migrant farmers; currently middle class

SPIRITUAL/RELIGIOUS

PHARMACOLOGIC

- Calcium
- Vitamins
- Hormone replacement
- Buspirone (BuSpar)

PSYCHOSOCIAL

- Impaired social isolation

LEGAL

ETHICAL

ALTERNATIVE THERAPY

- Herbal treatments containing Kava and Passaflora obtained from a curandara

PRIORITIZATION

DELEGATION

GENERALIZED ANXIETY DISORDER

Level of difficulty: Moderate

Overview: Requires critical thinking to understand and manage the common Hispanic practice of extended family being with a client for health care visits. The nurse must also identify behaviors common in clients with a diagnosis of Generalized Anxiety Disorder (GAD) and become knowledgeable about treatment modalities, including the antidepressant BuSpar.

Client Profile

Betty, a 50-year-old woman, came to this country with her parents when she was 7 years old. The family members worked as migrant farm workers until they had enough money to open a restaurant. Betty married young. She and her husband worked in the family restaurant and eventually bought it from the parents. They raised seven children, all grown and living on their own. Betty and her husband live in a mobile home close to the restaurant. She does not work in the family restaurant anymore because she worries excessively about doing a poor job. Betty no longer goes out if she can help it. She stays at home worrying about how she looks, what people think or say, the weather or road conditions, and many other things. Betty is not sleeping at night and keeps her husband awake when she roams the house. She keeps her clothing and belongings in perfect order while claiming she is doing a poor job of it. She does not prepare large family dinners anymore, though she still cooks the daily meals; one daughter has taken over the family dinners. This daughter has become concerned about Betty being isolated at home and worrying excessively and calls the community mental health center for an appointment for Betty.

Case Study

Betty presents at the community mental health center accompanied by her husband, her children and their spouses, several grandchildren, and a few cousins. When Betty's name is called and she is told that the nurse is ready to see her, she frowns and says: "What will I say? I don't know what to say. I think my slip is showing. My hem isn't straight."

Betty says she wants her whole family to go in to see the nurse with her. The nurse notices that Betty is extremely well groomed and dressed in spite of concerns she has been voicing about her appearance. Before the psychiatric nurse interviews Betty alone, she hears from the daughter that Betty "worries all the time" and although she has always been known to be a worrier, the worrying has become worse over the past six or eight months. The husband shares that his wife is keeping him awake at night with her inability to get to sleep or stay asleep.

The nurse interviews Betty alone. The nurse notices that Betty casts her eyes downward, speaks in a soft voice, does not smile, and seems restless as she taps her foot on the floor, drums her fingers on the table, and seems on the verge of getting out of her chair. Themes in the interview include: being tired, getting tired easily, not being able to concentrate, not getting work done, trouble sleeping, worrying about whether her husband loves her anymore and whether she and her husband have enough money, and not having the energy to attend to the housework or her clothing.

The nurse has the impression that Betty's anxiety floats from one worry to another. There is no convincing Betty that she looks all right. Any attempt to convince her that she need not worry about something in particular leads to a different worry before coming back to the earlier worry.

The community mental health psychiatrist examines Betty and, after a thorough physical examination and lab studies, finds nothing to explain her fatigue and difficulty sleeping other than anxiety. Betty produces her medicine bottles and says she is currently taking only vitamins, hormone replacement, and calcium. The psychiatrist asks the nurse to contact Betty's family health care provider to get information on any medical or psychiatric conditions he is treating her for; the report comes back that she has no medical diagnoses and the family health care provider thinks she suffers from anxiety. The psychiatrist prescribes buspirone (BuSpar) for Betty.

Two weeks later, during a home visit to Betty, the nurse learns, with some probing, that Betty is upset with her husband for loaning all their savings to the daughter and her husband to build a new home, while they continue to live in an older mobile home. At the end of the nurse's home visit, Betty's daughter arrives and tells the nurse that she wonders if Betty is making any progress. Betty also worries she is not getting better and asks the nurse about taking some herbal medicines containing Kava and Passaflora that her sister got from a curandara (folk healer); her sister wants to take her to see the curandara and have her do a ritual to cure the evil eye that was placed on Betty and made her sick.

Questions

1. What behaviors does this client have that match the criteria for a diagnosis of Generalized Anxiety Disorder?

2. How common is the diagnosis of Generalized Anxiety Disorder? Is it common for clients with GAD to have comorbidity, and should this client be assessed for any particular condition?

3. What explanation do you have for the number of family members coming to the community mental health center with this client? If you were the nurse, how would you deal with Betty's request for her whole family to accompany her to see you?

4. Before the nurse, or any other staff at the community mental health center, can talk with Betty's family health care provider, what do they need to do?

5. What does the nurse need to know about buspirone? What teaching needs to be done with the client in regard to buspirone? What medications other than buspirone are being used in the treatment of GAD, and how effective are they?

6. What are some of the interventions, in addition to antianxiety drugs, that are being used with clients who have GAD?

7. At one point the daughter says that she thinks Betty is not showing progress. What progress, if any, do you think has been made? What can you tell the daughter?

8. What do you think about Betty's sister using herbal remedies and rituals for driving out evil spirits in trying to cure Betty? Do herbal remedies work?

9. What nursing diagnoses would you write for Betty related to her Generalized Anxiety Disorder?

Caroline

GENDER

Female

AGE

19

SETTING

- Day treatment program in psychiatric hospital

ETHNICITY

- White American

CULTURAL CONSIDERATIONS

- Cajun, voodoo beliefs

PREEXISTING CONDITION

COEXISTING CONDITION

- Agoraphobia

COMMUNICATION

DISABILITY

SOCIOECONOMIC

SPIRITUAL/RELIGIOUS

- Voodoo

PHARMACOLOGIC

- Paroxetine (Paxil)

PSYCHOSOCIAL

LEGAL

ETHICAL

ALTERNATIVE THERAPY

PRIORITIZATION

DELEGATION

PANIC DISORDER WITH AGORAPHOBIA

Level of difficulty: High

Overview: Requires the nurse to develop an understanding of Agoraphobia and Panic Disorder and to use critical thinking to teach the client ways to minimize symptoms of a panic attack and overcome a fear of leaving her house. The nurse must also help a client's peers understand that voodoo beliefs can be cultural practices, not psychosis.

DIFFICULT

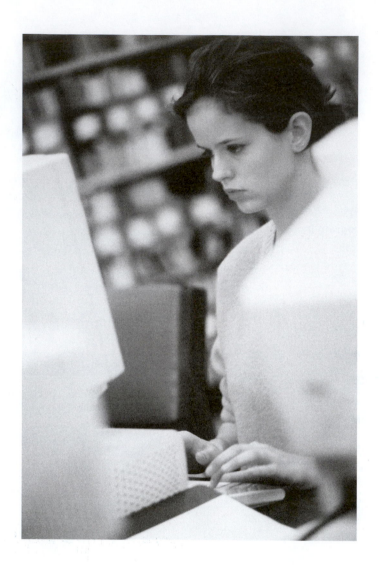

Client Profile

Caroline, a 19-year-old college student from rural Louisiana, is attending a large university in a nearby state. Caroline was doing well at the university until she experienced several unexpected panic attacks. She had a panic attack in the undergraduate library and another one when she went to the gym to work out. The most recent attack occurred about a month ago when she was driving her car. Suddenly and for no reason she could think of, she began feeling short of breath. It "felt like someone was smothering" her, but she was alone in the car. She was afraid she was going to die. Her heart was going very fast; she became dizzy and was feeling numbness and tingling in her hands. She felt a sense of impending danger and wanting to escape. She was so panicked that she had to pull over into a convenience store parking lot and wait until she felt better to call her boyfriend and ask him to come and take her home.

Caroline rode the bus to campus to classes for a while after this panic attack. She parked her car and refused to drive anywhere. She began fearing another panic attack and started skipping classes. A big school football game and party is coming up, and the boyfriend threatens to break up with Caroline if she does not "get a grip."

Case Study

Caroline's mother receives a call from Caroline's roommate telling her of the situation. Her mother takes Caroline to see a psychiatrist who prescribes paroxetine (Paxil) 10 mg/day and suggests an outpatient evening treatment program. Treatment in the evening allows Caroline to go to classes in the daytime. Caroline attends the first two nights of group and individual therapy. Her mother drives Caroline to the evening program on these nights. During group therapy Caroline reveals a fear that she has some life-threatening illness that the doctor has not found on a recent annual physical. Later in group she says she thinks someone has put a voodoo spell on her.

On the third night, Caroline is to take a cab or bus to the evening sessions because her mother has gone back home. It is two hours before the evening program is to begin. Caroline calls the nurse in the outpatient evening treatment program, saying: "I am too afraid to leave the house. I'm sorry. I just can't come tonight. Perhaps I will be able to come tomorrow." The nurse responds, "I want you to take several deep breaths and think about relaxing. Now that you feel very relaxed, I want you to visualize in your mind walking to the door and opening it."

Questions

1. What is the difference between a panic attack and Panic Disorder? What symptoms does Caroline have, and do they match the criteria for a diagnosis of Panic Disorder?

2. What is the usual onset of panic attacks and Panic Disorder? Is there a gender difference in the prevalence of panic attacks and Panic Disorder?

3. Caroline has Agoraphobia. What is Agoraphobia and what symptoms of this problem does Caroline exhibit?

4. How can Caroline's significant others (e.g., mother, boyfriend, roommate, classmates, and peers in group) best support her in dealing with panic attacks and Agoraphobia?

5. One of Caroline's group peers shares with the nurse that he thinks Caroline is psychotic and is paranoid and delusional about somebody putting a spell on her. If you were the nurse, how would you respond?

6. How would you respond if Caroline shares with you that she believes she has a fatal disease that no one has found and that someone is putting a spell on her or choking and putting pins in a voodoo doll that represents her?

7. Why did the nurse respond by encouraging relaxation and visualization when Caroline called to say she would not make it to the evening therapy program?

8. What teaching does the nurse need to do with Caroline in regard to the paroxetine (Paxil) she has begun to take for her Panic Disorder? What problem associated with paroxetine (Paxil) often causes clients, particularly men, to stop taking it, and what can be done about this? What assessments does the nurse need to do because Caroline is on paroxetine (Paxil)?

9. What medications have been found to be effective in reducing the number and/or severity of panic attacks?

10. What therapies other than medication are currently being used to treat Panic Disorder and Agoraphobia?

11. What nursing diagnoses would you write for Caroline?

12. Discuss some nursing interventions for at least one of the likely nursing diagnoses.

13. Carolyn's boyfriend asks: "What causes Panic Disorder?" How would you answer him? Why might he be concerned?

GENDER	**SPIRITUAL/RELIGIOUS**
Female	
AGE	**PHARMACOLOGIC**
25	■ Trazodone (Desyrl)
SETTING	**PSYCHOSOCIAL**
■ General hospital	■ Impaired social interaction
ETHNICITY	■ Situational low self-esteem
■ Central American	**LEGAL**
CULTURAL CONSIDERATIONS	■ Confidentiality
■ Colombian	■ Consent for release of information
PREEXISTING CONDITION	**ETHICAL**
	■ Client's right not to report a crime vs. nurse and health care team members' views
COEXISTING CONDITION	**ALTERNATIVE THERAPY**
COMMUNICATION	**PRIORITIZATION**
DISABILITY	**DELEGATION**
SOCIOECONOMIC	

POST TRAUMATIC STRESS DISORDER (PTSD), ADULT

Level of difficulty: High

Overview: Requires the nurse to select therapeutic communication techniques to use with a client who has signs and symptoms of PTSD. The nurse must decide what action to take when the client reveals being raped in the past and asks the nurse to keep this information confidential. The nurse is challenged to do holistic nursing with this client who has psychological needs and sexual education and support needs as well as medical needs.

Client Profile

Claudia is a single, bright 25-year-old graduate student from a small town in the mountains of Colombia in Central America. She came to the United States to do her graduate work at a large state university. One night she decided to go meet friends at a local bar frequented by college students, locals, and tourists. Her friends did not show up. A nice-looking man bought her a few drinks and then offered to take her home. When she arrived home this man forcibly performed sexual acts and made her perform sexual acts on him. He then forced her to shower to "wash away evidence" and threatened to kill her if she reported the incident. She felt a great deal of fear and helplessness. Claudia thought perhaps this rape was her fault for dressing too sexy or going out unescorted. Almost immediately Claudia began to have a feeling of being numb and detached from everything and seemed to be in a daze, and she seemed to not be able to recall much of the incident at all. She continued her studies and moved in with her boyfriend, but did not tell him about the incident, and she has not told her family in Colombia that she has moved in with her boyfriend. She avoided the bar and the friends that she was supposed to meet. She decided she would move on with her life.

Eventually she started having trouble falling asleep and had nightmares, and her boyfriend recognized she was less interested in intimacy and had begun talking about never getting married or having children. She asked him not to wear a certain aftershave, which she had always complimented him on before.

Case Study

About a year after the rape episode, Claudia is admitted to the general hospital for an appendectomy. The night after surgery Claudia screams in the middle of the night and the night nurse finds her crying. The night nurse decides to sit with Claudia until she relaxes. The nurse offers to sit with Claudia and to listen if she wants to talk and then sits quietly.

Claudia is silent for a while, and then says: "I have had bad dreams almost every night for about a year, and I have bad memories come on me sometimes in the daytime. I have not told anyone about it, and I don't want to talk about it, but I was raped about a year ago and please do not put that in my chart. I am here to have surgery and not talk about the rape. That is in the past. Even my boyfriend does not know about it." The nurse notices that Claudia is hypervigilant, alert to every small noise and is easily startled.

Two days later, the health care provider gives Claudia a tentative diagnosis of Post Traumatic Stress Disorder (PTSD) and asks a psychiatric mental health nurse clinician employed by the hospital to work with the client and the medical team.

Questions

1. What communication techniques did the night nurse use that encouraged the client to reveal that her bad dreams had to do with being raped? Were these recognized therapeutic communication techniques? What other therapeutic communication techniques could the nurse use in response to the client saying she was raped a few months ago?

2. If you were the night nurse and the client asked you not to tell anyone about the rape, how would you respond, and what would you do with the information?

3. The client promises you she will talk with her doctor in the morning. What could you chart about the client's crying out?

4. If the client were to agree to let you call the health care provider in the middle of the night, what would you say to this provider?

Questions (continued)

5. The client is talking about the rape being all her fault for not using better judgment and dressing provocatively. Is this unusual behavior from a rape victim? How do you, as her nurse, respond?

6. Do you pass on this information about the client saying she had been raped in the report to the next shift? What sort of things do you consider in making your decision?

7. Looking at the information in the client profile and the case study, what signs and symptoms has this client had, and perhaps still has, that led the health care provider to a tentative diagnosis of PTSD? If diagnosed with PTSD, would this client likely be diagnosed as having acute, chronic, or delayed onset PTSD?

8. What events can place individuals at risk for PTSD, and which events have the highest risk?

9. What nursing diagnoses would you write for this client, given the limited amount of information that you have?

10. What are some of the current treatments for PTSD?

11. What teaching would you do about trazodone (Desyrl) with this client?

12. How can the primary nurse work with the client in regard to sexuality? How can the primary nurse teach the boyfriend ways to be supportive as well as to deal with his expressed concerns about the client's decreased interest in sexual intimacy?

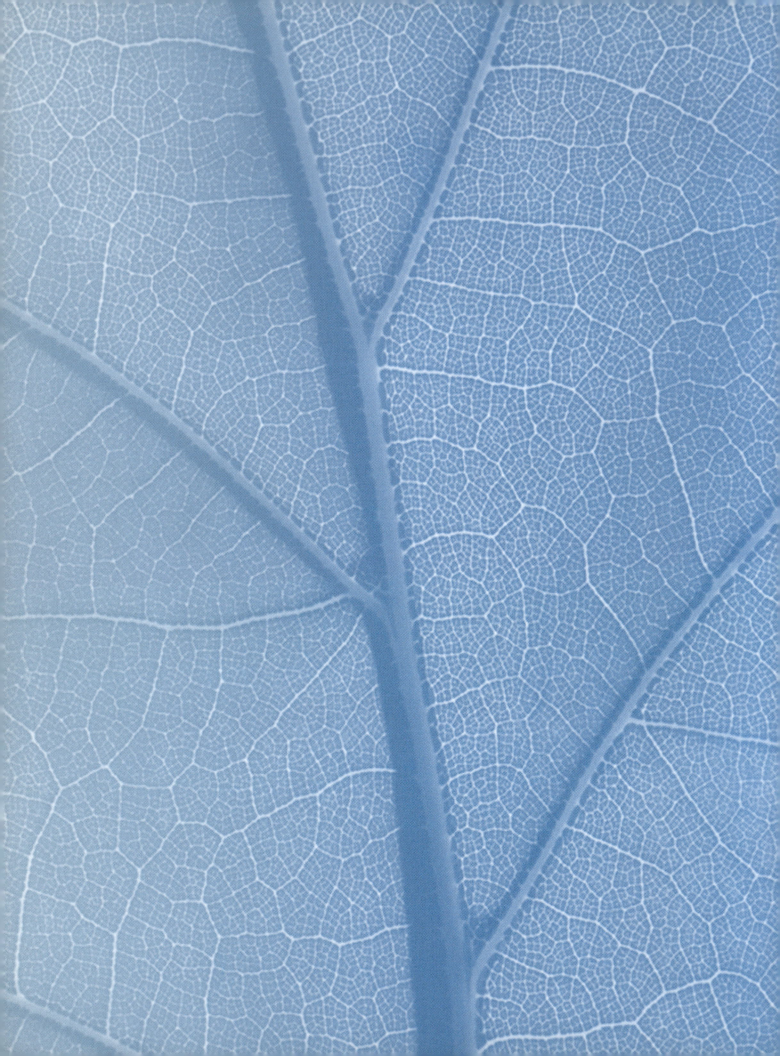

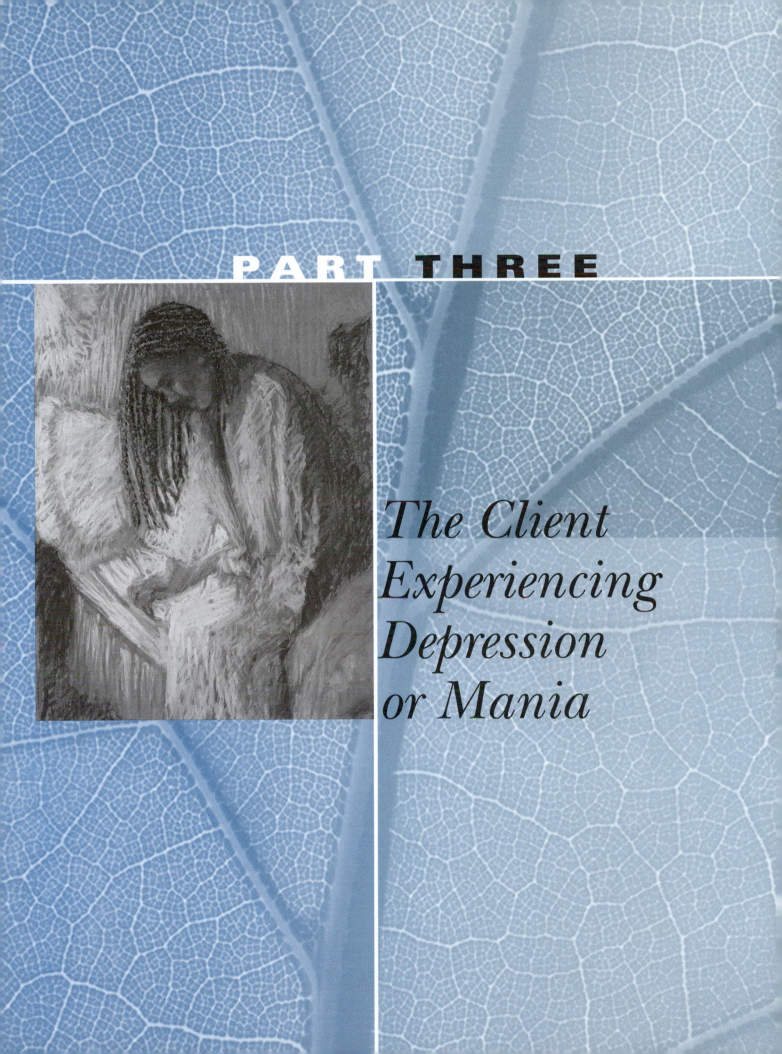

PART THREE

The Client Experiencing Depression or Mania

GENDER

Male

AGE

14

SETTING

- Adolescent unit of a psychiatric hospital

ETHNICITY

- Black American

CULTURAL CONSIDERATIONS

PREEXISTING CONDITION

COEXISTING CONDITION

- Obesity Hypoventilation Syndrome

COMMUNICATION

DISABILITY

SOCIOECONOMIC

- Low-income family
- Public assistance
- Housing project

SPIRITUAL/RELIGIOUS

PHARMACOLOGIC

- Vitamins
- Sertraline (Zoloft)

PSYCHOSOCIAL

- Social relationships with peers limited due to obesity/depressed mood
- Low self-esteem

LEGAL

- Obtaining permission for a child or adolescent to take an antidepressant

ETHICAL

- Alternative therapy

PRIORITIZATION

- Addressing physical and psychological conditions while acknowledging self-esteem and identity-building needs

DELEGATION

- Delegation of crisis on unit to another team member

DYSTHYMIA

Level of difficulty: Easy

Overview: Requires the nurse to build a trusting relationship with a young client and his mother. The nurse must determine whether to respond to a unit crisis or delegate that task to a nurse colleague, so a promise to the client and mother can be kept. Challenges for the nurse also include making the mother part of the team identifying treatment goals and interventions. The nurse is called upon to describe current theories of treatment of dysthymia and to demonstrate understanding of a coexisting physical problem: Obesity Hypoventilation Syndrome.

Client Profile

John is a 14-year-old male who lives in urban public housing with his mother. John's father is not in contact. John has had a low level of energy and is described by his mother and teachers as looking sad and being somewhat irritable for the past eighteen months. His major activities outside of school are watching television, using the computer, eating, and attending the native Baptist Church with his mother. Peers in the housing project make fun of John for attending church with his mother, but he likes the church music and the church potluck suppers.

John resists joining activities. He declines peer activity and offers one or more reasons why the activity is not desirable. "I don't care" is a phrase he frequently uses (e.g., if he doesn't do his homework and is given a consequence, he says: "I don't care"). His teachers describe John as "easily distracted" unless he is doing something he is extremely interested in. He is morbidly obese and short of breath after walking a short distance. John is found on a routine school physical to be somewhat depressed and so overweight that it affects his breathing. The health care provider doing the physical refers John to an endocrinologist and a psychiatrist.

Case Study

John is admitted to the adolescent unit of a private psychiatric hospital by his endocrinologist and psychiatrist. The hospital is interested in receiving additional future admissions with similar psychiatric diagnoses and endocrine problems combined, and agrees to accept this case without payment.

On admission, the admitting nurse greets the client and his mother and introduces himself. The nurse interviews John's mother while John is given a tour of the unit. During the interview, a staff member comes and asks the admitting nurse to step out to discuss something urgent. The nurse tells John's mother he will be right back. The staff nurse describes an urgent situation on the unit and indicates the admitting nurse should take care of it; however, the admitting nurse delegates it to someone else and returns quickly to continue the interview. The mother is asked to describe a typical day in the family in chronological sequence and to write down what she and John had eaten at meals the previous day. Later, when the nurse interviews John alone, he asks John: "What do you like to do that you are good at?" John replies: "I can cook, do really cool magic tricks, and play computer games." John tells the nurse that other kids are mean to him and tell him he is too fat to play with them. He says he would like to be able to play football. John is shown a page of faces with various expressions and asked to pick out the way he feels most of the time. He picks out the sad face.

Just before mother leaves, she says to the nurse: "John's birthday is next week; I want to bring a birthday cake for him. Would that be all right if I brought a second cake for the other kids?"

John's tentative diagnoses are early onset Dysthymic Disorder and Obesity Hypoventilation Syndrome. He is admitted for professional help in safely losing weight, to begin medication for dysthymia, and to participate in group, family, and individual therapy. In addition to orders for these therapies, the admission orders include daily vitamins and a strict diet (e.g., protein diet drink to be mixed by the nutritionist and sent to the unit three times a day, one cup of salad, and a four-ounce skinless broiled chicken breast or broiled piece of fish at lunch and dinner). The orders also include nocturnal polysomnography testing in the sleep studies laboratory. Oxygen saturation levels are to be taken four times a day, and John is to wear a pulse oxymeter at night and recordings of the readings are to be made every hour. A $PaCO_2$ level is to be drawn during the day. In the progress notes, the health care provider writes: "Consider Sertraline (Zoloft)."

Questions

1. Discuss how John's observed behavior may or may not match a diagnosis of Dysthymic Disorder (DD). How do the criteria for a diagnosis of DD differ for adults compared to children and adolescents? What does the psychiatrist mean when he refers to John as having early onset Dysthymic Disorder (EODD)?

2. What is the risk for a person in a clinical setting with a diagnosis of Dysthymic Disorder to develop a major depressive disorder?

3. Is ethnicity a risk factor for Dysthymic Disorder? Are there other risk factors? What gender differences, if any, are there in the occurrence of Dysthymic Disorder in children and in adults?

4. Describe the usual course of Dysthymic Disorder.

5. Discuss what you know about Obesity Hypoventilation Syndrome from your reading on this subject.

6. When the staff member called the nurse out of the interview with John's mother, why do you suppose he delegated whatever needed doing and went right back into the interview?

7. The nurse asked John what he likes to do and what he is good at. What can the nurse and the treatment team use this information for?

8. Describe the possible reasons for John to go to individual, group, and family therapy sessions.

9. If you were the admitting nurse and John's mother asked you if she could bring him a birthday cake the following week, what would your response be?

10. From the limited information you have been given, what nursing diagnoses are most likely for this client?

11. Describe some interventions you would use for at least one of these nursing diagnoses.

12. What is the health care provider likely considering before starting sertraline (Zoloft)? What assessments need to be done prior to the client being started on sertraline, and what teaching needs to be done with the client and the client's mother? Who needs to sign permission for the client to take sertraline?

Maria

GENDER

Female

AGE

35

SETTING

- Inpatient hospital psychiatric unit

ETHNICITY

- Central American

CULTURAL CONSIDERATIONS

- Hispanic culture, rural Nicaraguan

PREEXISTING CONDITION

COEXISTING CONDITION

COMMUNICATION

- Speaks little English; Spanish preferred language

DISABILITY

SOCIOECONOMIC

- Raised by poor parents; now upper middle class

SPIRITUAL/RELIGIOUS

- Catholic

PHARMACOLOGIC

- Birth control
- Lithium carbonate (Eskalith)
- Olanzapine (Zyprexa)

PSYCHOSOCIAL

LEGAL

- Confidentiality
- Right to refuse medication

ETHICAL

- Birth control vs. Catholic teachings

ALTERNATIVE THERAPY

PRIORITIZATION

DELEGATION

- collaborating treatment planning with team
- collaborating management of lithium levels with team

BIPOLAR I MANIC EPISODE

Level of difficulty: Moderate

Overview: Requires critical thinking to therapeutically deal with the client's lack of judgment in areas such as spending, sexuality, and dress. Requires the nurse to consider how a client's culture and religion can affect treatment. The client's high levels of energy, activity, and distractibility require the nurse to develop strategies to get the client to eat, sleep, and attend to hygiene tasks. Requires management of the client's medication at a therapeutic level and to delegate this aspect of care at discharge.

Client Profile

Maria is a 35-year-old married female born and raised in a small village in Nicaragua, Central America. Her parents are poor. Her husband is a university professor who was serving as a Peace Corps worker when they met. She has been in the United States for two years and speaks a little English but requires Spanish for clear understanding. They have a 4-year-old daughter. Maria has been diagnosed with Bipolar I and takes lithium carbonate. Recently she stopped taking her lithium and has been staying up all night and eating very little. She is dressing and behaving in a sexually provocative manner and going on spending sprees buying things she does not need and cannot afford (e.g., a motorcycle that she does not know how to ride and a drum set that she does not know how to play). Her husband decides she is out of control and calls Maria's psychiatrist who suggests admission to the psychiatric unit of the hospital.

Case Study

During the admission process, the nurse observes that Maria is dressed in a short and tight-fitting dress. Her speech is clear but sprinkled with profanity as she moves rapidly from topic to topic. At the nurse's request, Maria sits down, then jumps up and moves about the room.

Maria's husband says that Maria has stopped taking her lithium and has not been sleeping or eating enough. He describes her extravagant purchases, some of which were returned or given away to strangers (e.g., Maria gave part of a drum set to a man she met in a bar). The husband explains that Maria has put the family in serious debt and states she is unfit to care for their child. With her husband translating for her, Maria objects to being admitted to the hospital, but then agrees to admission. The husband expresses concern about her sexually provocative behavior and states he fears that she will get sexually involved with other clients.

At the first meal after admission, Maria is in the dining room with the other clients. Instead of eating, Maria carries napkins to, and talks to, all the other clients and ignores the food. Staff members have told Maria several times to sit down and eat, and she has not complied.

The nurse asks the dietitian to prepare a sandwich and a banana for Maria. After the clients are finished with lunch, the nurse suggests Maria go to her room to wash her face and hands.

The psychiatrist-ordered pregnancy test comes back negative. The psychiatrist orders Lithium carbonate (Eskalith), olanzapine (Zyprexa), and birth control pills.

At medication time, the nurse gives Maria her medications and then examines Maria's mouth. The nurse does some teaching about the medications with Maria, who becomes upset when she learns she has been prescribed birth control and says she will not take it as it is not allowed in her religion.

The nurse notices that Maria is irritable and verbally hostile at times as well as inappropriate during her first days on the unit. During one encounter with Maria, the nurse senses great hostile energy coming from Maria, who says, "You think you so smart! You don't know nothing!" Sometimes Maria is demanding or threatening. For example, she demands that the nurse send someone to the store to pick up items for her and take her credit card to pay for them. Maria continues to dress and talk in a sexually provocative manner. She asks the male nurse, who passes medications in the early morning, to perform some sexual acts with her. At one point Maria is intrusive with another client in the day room and the client is threatening to harm Maria. The nurse observes that both clients are loud and their behavior is escalating.

After one month, during a meeting of the psychiatric health team, the psychiatrist discusses Maria's past psychiatric history, which includes two episodes of depression and one of mania. He offers a diagnosis of Bipolar I, Manic Episode for Maria. He orders that blood be drawn for a lithium level. The lithium level comes back at 1.5.

Questions

1. What criteria is essential for a diagnosis of Bipolar I? What would need to be different for Maria to have a diagnosis of Bipolar II Disorder? Which of Maria's behaviors are consistent with the criteria for a manic episode?

2. What would it feel like to be manic, and why would someone who is manic stop taking medication to bring their mood down to "normal"?

3. If you were Maria's nurse, what needs would you assess in relation to her culture and communication? What accommodations would you most likely try to make for her?

4. Why did the nurse ask the dietitian to prepare a sandwich and a banana for Maria, and why did the nurse take Maria to her room?

5. What is the most likely reason for the psychiatrist ordering a pregnancy test on admission? Why did he order birth control pills? The client has refused the birth control pills. How do you feel about this, and what action would you take if you were the nurse in this case?

6. What reason did the nurse have for inspecting Maria's mouth after giving her the medication?

7. What teaching did the nurse need to do about lithium for Maria? What is the significance of the lithium level, and what action(s) does the nurse need to take, if any?

8. What is olanzapine (Zyprexa), and what is the likely reason that Maria is being prescribed olanzapine?

9. What would you do or say if you were the nurse standing in front of Maria when she says: "You think you so smart. You don't know nothing"?

10. What strategies could a nurse use when Maria is demanding that a staff member be sent to shop for her using her credit card? Do strategies differ depending on whether the client has supportive family and/or friends, or not?

11. What might you say or do in response to the husband's expressed fear that his wife will become involved sexually with a peer on the unit?

12. How would you feel and what would you say or do if you were the male nurse passing medications and Maria was talking seductively and using profanity?

13. When the nurse finds Maria has been intrusive with another client and that both clients are escalating and threatening, what is the best response by the nurse?

14. What are some potential nursing diagnoses that you could likely write for this client?

15. What developmental stage is Maria in, and what behaviors, if any, does she have to match the tasks of this stage?

CASE STUDY 3

Candice

GENDER

Female

AGE

13

SETTING

- Adolescent unit of private psychiatric hospital

ETHNICITY

- White American

CULTURAL CONSIDERATIONS

PREEXISTING CONDITION

COEXISTING CONDITION

- Marijuana use

COMMUNICATION

DISABILITY

SOCIOECONOMIC

- Upper class; has trust fund

SPIRITUAL/RELIGIOUS

PHARMACOLOGIC

PSYCHOSOCIAL

LEGAL

ETHICAL

ALTERNATIVE THERAPY

PRIORITIZATION

- Prioritizing urgent vs. important tasks

DELEGATION

- Delegating to mental health technician

MOOD DISORDER IN A CHILD, BIPOLAR EPISODE

Level of difficulty: Moderate

Overview: Requires critical thinking to determine least restrictive yet effective interventions with an adolescent who has a family history of Bipolar Disorder (BPD) and symptoms of a Manic Episode. Requires therapeutic communication skills as well as empathy to help the client's parents understand treatment approaches and feel they are an essential part of the treatment team. Requires an understanding of the basic principles involved in seclusion and restraint.

Client Profile

Candice is a 13-year-old female whose grandfather made a fortune in the oil business and left her a trust fund when he died. Her grandfather was known to have required little sleep and to have a phenomenal amount of energy at times. He was said to have had a number of mistresses, sometimes gone on spending sprees, and given extravagant tips to waitresses even when he only ordered a cup of coffee. Once when he was in a private psychiatric hospital, he ordered two hundred steak dinners and called a taxi to pick them up and deliver them to the hospital for all the patients and staff. He called a jeweler and ordered a diamond ring for one of the nurses he had just met and then threatened to get five lawyers to come to the hospital when she refused to marry him. Grandfather eventually committed suicide, but not before he was diagnosed as manic-depressive (term used before Bipolar Disorder came into use) and put on lithium, which he refused to take.

Candice recently has been having a somewhat elated mood (e.g., giggling about things that others don't find funny and taking about the exquisite beauty in mundane things such as a light bulb). The speed of her speech has increased, and she jumps rapidly from topic to topic. She has been staying up all night drawing original cartoons and/or rearranging her room and the family living room. At school, Candice has recently been going to the principal's office or catching her in the hall to tell her how to run the school better. She also tells the teacher how to make the classroom better. At school Candice was caught kissing a boy in the boy's restroom and the teacher intercepted a note that Candice wrote to another boy suggesting they engage in sex. Candice's father discovered that she was e-mailing a 27-year-old man that she had never met and planned to run away with him. She denied drug use but admitted that she had started smoking cigarettes and occasionally smoked marijuana, which she had gotten from her father's desk. Candice's father had her evaluated by a child-adolescent psychiatrist, and she was admitted to the adolescent unit of a private psychiatric hospital for evaluation and treatment. Candice's parents were worried that they could not keep Candice from running away and getting into trouble so they agreed to pay whatever it cost.

Case Study

Candice has been admitted to the adolescent unit. The nurse notices that Candice is pacing rapidly in the day room and goes to talk to her. Candice talks rapidly, moving from topic to topic. One of her themes is getting out of the hospital to meet her "friend." As the nurse walks away, she hears one of Candice's peers on the unit tell her: "Back off; get out of my face." The nurse then sees Candice scratching and hitting the peer. When a male mental health technician tries to pull Candice away from the peer, Candice scratches him deeply with her long fingernails and kicks him. Other staff members, including the nurse, take Candice to the seclusion room. The nurse calls the psychiatrist for an order to seclude Candice, who is in the seclusion room scratching herself superficially with her nails and smearing blood on the walls. The mental health worker reports later that Candice is asleep in the seclusion room. When she awakes the nurse talks with her and decides to let her out of seclusion but not before cutting Candice's fingernails. When Candice's parents come to visit, they are very angry about her long nails being cut and about her being put in seclusion. They express concern about the possibility of sexual activity with boys on the unit and whether or not Candice is stopping her seemingly constant motion long enough to eat.

MOOD LOG

Name: _____   Month: _____   Year: _____

Rate mood

0 ———— 50 ———— 100
Dep   Normal   Mania

Days of Month →	1	2	3	4	5	6	7	8	9	10	11	12	13	14	15	16	17	18	19	20	21	22	23	24	25	26	27	28	29	30	31
Mania																															
Depression																															
Anxiety (1–10)																															

Medication

	1	2	3	4	5	6	7	8	9	10	11	12	13	14	15	16	17	18	19	20	21	22	23	24	25	26	27	28	29	30	31
Menses																															
Sleep																															

A mood log can be used to document periods of mania and depression

Questions

1. Should you, if you were the nurse in this case, have gotten an order from the physician before secluding the client? When secluding a client, is it ever correct to delegate all communication with the client to another team member such as a mental health technician?

2. Discuss safety precautions and tasks required of the staff when a child or adolescent is secluded. What needs to be documented? How would you decide when to release the client from seclusion?

3. Just as you pick up the phone to call the health care provider for orders for secluding Candice, another adolescent client comes running up to you and says: "I need to talk with you right now about something very important." Do you stop what you are doing and listen, get the orders first then listen, send this child to another staff member, or come up with another solution?

4. After the client is out of seclusion, you sit in on a debriefing with the seclusion team. Do you think that the situation in the day room that led to seclusion was handled well, or could seclusion have been avoided? Could the injuries have been avoided? What would you say or do in the briefing?

5. What behaviors do children and adolescents who are diagnosed with Bipolar Disorder exhibit? What diagnostic criteria would Candice, or other children and/or adolescents, have to meet to be diagnosed as having a Bipolar Episode or a Bipolar Disorder? Does her behavior match any of these criteria?

6. Describe why clinicians have difficulty diagnosing mood disorders in children and adolescents and why parents and clinicians confuse it with other disorders.

7. What do you think causes Bipolar Disorder? Does genetics play a role in the cause of Bipolar Disorder? What is the age of onset and the usual course of Bipolar Disorder? Is the course the same in children compared to adults?

8. What is your response to the parents' anger about Candice being in seclusion and having her nails cut? How would you answer the parents in regard to their concerns about their daughter's possible sexual activity while in the facility?

9. What nursing diagnoses are you likely to write for this client given what information you have? What are some tentative goals that you might develop with input from the client/family/colleagues on the unit? What interventions do you think would be necessary and/or helpful?

10. What medications and treatments are being used today for children and adolescents who are exhibiting signs of mood disorders, particularly signs of a Bipolar Disorder?

11. What research has been done, or is currently being carried out, with children and adolescents who have a diagnosis of Bipolar Disorder?

Elke

GENDER

Female

AGE

41

SETTING

- Psychiatric unit of a general hospital

ETHNICITY

- German

CULTURAL CONSIDERATIONS

- German
- Military

PREEXISTING CONDITION

COEXISTING CONDITION

COMMUNICATION

DISABILITY

SOCIOECONOMIC

SPIRITUAL/RELIGIOUS

PHARMACOLOGIC

- Citalopram hydrochloride (Celexa)

PSYCHOSOCIAL

- Isolating

LEGAL

- Confidentiality
- Client right to refuse treatment

ETHICAL

- Respect for confidentiality vs. informing neighbor to ensure client safely.

ALTERNATIVE THERAPY

PRIORITIZATION

- Safety issues

DELEGATION

MAJOR DEPRESSIVE DISORDER

Level of difficulty: High

Overview: Requires the nurse to identify symptoms of major depression, look at factors contributing to depression, and identify strategies to prevent suicide.

DIFFICULT

Client Profile

Elke, a 41-year-old female, came to the United States five years ago, shortly after marrying a career U.S. military soldier. Elke has two children: a 10-year-old from a previous marriage and a 6-year-old from the current marriage. Elke has been a meticulous housekeeper and has managed the family finances. Since arriving in the United States, she has not been back to Germany to see her parents and siblings. Although she would very much like to visit her family, she can't afford to do so.

Case Study

Elke is admitted to the psychiatric unit of the city's general hospital. Her husband had noticed that she was so depressed she no longer laughed or smiled. She had admitted to him that she had been having thoughts of killing herself. She was not eating or drinking enough, had lost fifteen pounds in three weeks, and was not attending to her hygiene. Elke seemed to have little or no interest in anything except sleeping or sitting in a chair. The client's husband accompanies her on admission and shares with the staff that he is afraid Elke will kill herself and he is unable to watch her around the clock. He says that he believes if she does not kill herself by some means such as hoarding pills and overdosing that she will deteriorate by not eating or drinking enough.

On admission the psychiatric nurse asks Elke about any prior episodes of depression. The client admits to having had a deep depression about a year prior. The nurse assesses Elke for suicide ideation and finds her describing feeling like she is in a deep dark hole with no way out and her life is hopeless. The nurse first assesses the client alone and then talks with the husband and client. At one point the nurse asks Elke to tell her what it means when someone says: "Don't cry over spilled milk." Elke says: "Don't cry when milk is spilled because you can buy some more at the store."

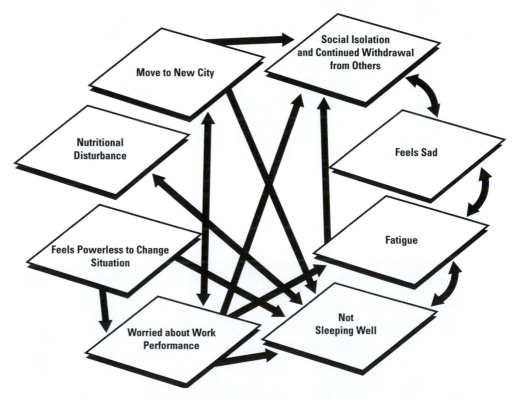

Concept map of issues and problems associated with depression

The nurse takes Elke's vital signs, weight, and height. Her vital signs are normal: height is 5 foot 5 inches and weight is 100 pounds.

The psychiatrist puts Elke on citalopram hydrochloride (Celexa), an SSRI. The nurse who admits Elke, and who continues to be assigned to her, notices that Elke isolates, verbalizes very little, and does little except when she is prompted and rewarded with points. Elke refuses to play volleyball or go to the movies with peers and staff. About five weeks after admission, Elke seems to be doing better. Her affect is brighter. She begins to play the piano in the dayroom. She asks the doctor for a pass to go home briefly to pay some bills and check on things there. Her children are now at her mother-in-law's home and her husband is away on military duty, and she has to take care of paying the bills.

Questions

1. Which signs and symptoms does Elke have that are consistent with those of a Major Depressive Episode?

2. What factor(s) do you think could have contributed to Elke's depression?

3. Why is the nurse interested in whether Elke has had prior episodes of major depression?

4. The nurse makes an observation that Elke had an episode of depression one year ago. What does the nurse need to learn from Elke and/or her husband, and what significance could it possibly have if Elke were depressed every year at the same time?

5. Why does the nurse ask Elke to interpret what is meant by "Don't cry over spilled milk"? What does the nurse learn from Elke's response?

6. What percentage of people with Major Depressive Disorder kill themselves? What could the nurse do to help keep Elke from killing herself?

7. How would you feel if you were Elke, and what would you need if you were Elke? What would it be like to be Elke's spouse or to be the spouse of any person with Major Depressive Disorder?

8. What interventions would you most likely initiate if you were writing a care plan for someone like Elke?

9. When Elke's mood seems to improve greatly and she wants to get a pass to go home and take care of some urgent business, would you support her having a pass? Why or why not?

10. The health care provider signs the pass allowing Elke to go home for four hours, provided an adult accompanies her, and she gets her neighbor to drive her home and back. What would you do if you were Elke's nurse?

11. What is a token economy or a point system, and how is this used to change behavior?

12. Is ECT used today for clients with depression? How do you feel about this?

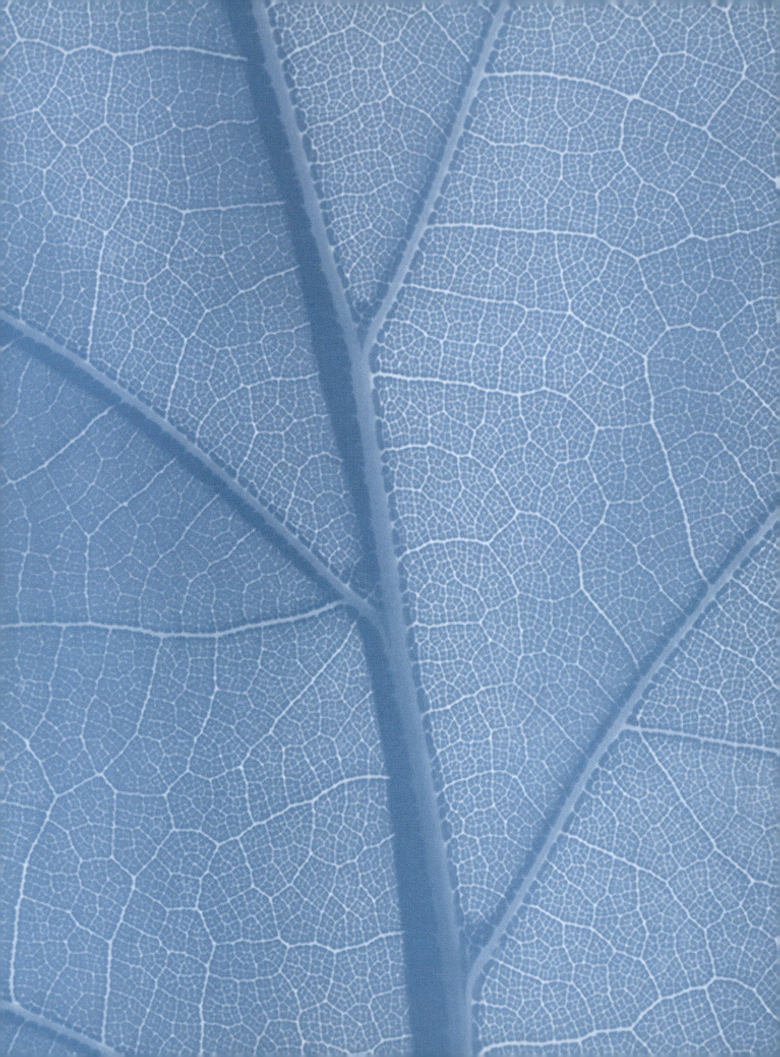

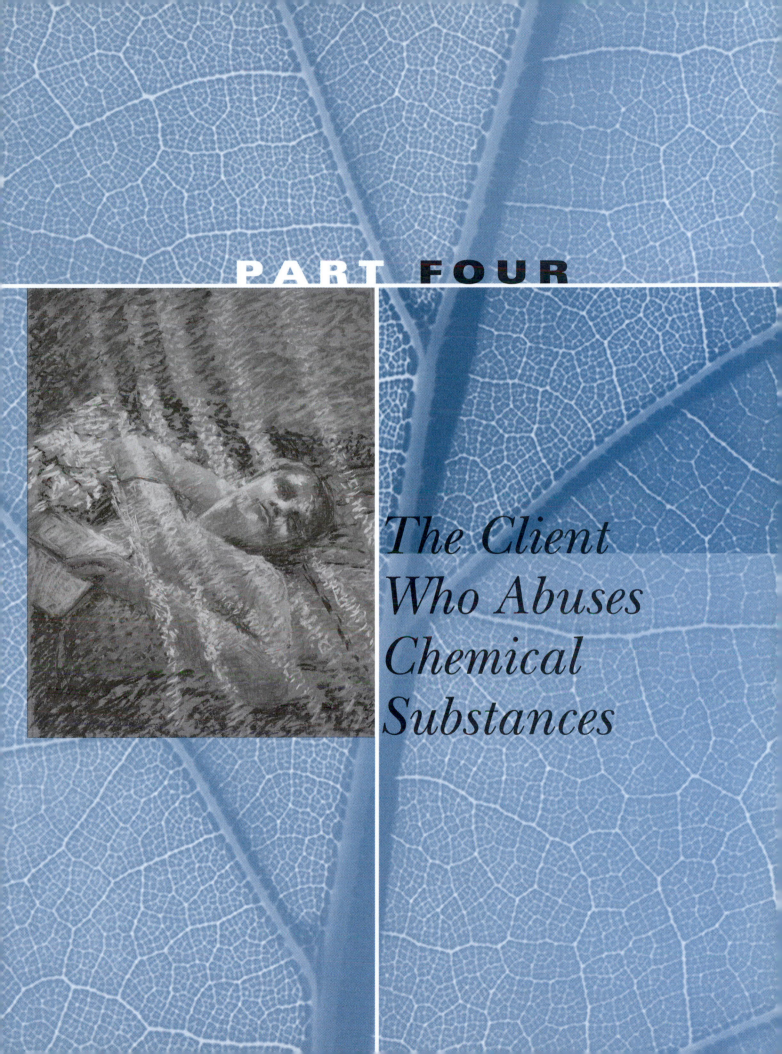

PART FOUR

The Client Who Abuses Chemical Substances

Ron

GENDER

Male

AGE

42

SETTING

- Hospital

ETHNICITY

- White American

CULTURAL CONSIDERATIONS

- "Hippie" culture

PREEXISTING CONDITION

COEXISTING CONDITION

COMMUNICATION

DISABILITY

SOCIOECONOMIC

- Middle class

SPIRITUAL/RELIGIOUS

- Buddhist

PHARMACOLOGIC

PSYCHOSOCIAL

LEGAL

- Illegal drug possession and use
- Charting must be factual
- Possibility of nurse involvement in court proceedings

ETHICAL

- Care based on client lifestyle

ALTERNATIVE THERAPY

- Acupuncture

PRIORITIZATION

DELEGATION

MODERATE

CANNABIS ABUSE

Level of difficulty: Moderate

Overview: This case involves treating an illegal drug user with additional health concerns.

Client Profile

Ron is a 42-year-old high school teacher who smokes marijuana (Cannabis sativa) occasionally. He has been using marijuana with varying intensity since junior high school. His drug use prolonged his college education, but he did eventually earn a bachelor's degree and teaching certificate for high-school-level history, English, and science. The drug use also contributed to the dissolution of his first marriage. Since then he has become fascinated with Buddhist teachings and studies them often.

Ron continues to smoke marijuana "to relax," although it makes him anxious, paranoid, and impacts his short-term memory. He has to be particularly careful that none of his students or their parents see him, so he only smokes at his home or the homes of close friends, and never within several hours of teaching. The school has a zero tolerance policy on drug use.

After an argument, Ron's girlfriend, Patsy, hid some marijuana in his briefcase and then anonymously notified the principal of his school once Ron had gone to work. Due to the tip, the principal inspected Ron's briefcase, found the marijuana, and notified the police. Ron was suspended from his job, but after Patsy admitted to planting the marijuana, the school board agreed to give Ron another chance if he would complete a twenty-eight-day (two weeks inpatient and two weeks outpatient) treatment program and agree to abstain from marijuana or other illegal substance use following treatment. Ron consented to save his job. He has a court date in a month for a charge of marijuana possession.

Case Study

Ron decides to smoke a little marijuana to control his nerves and mellow himself out before going to be admitted to the drug treatment program. He also reasons that he should smoke the remainder of his marijuana rather than flush it down the toilet. On the way to the program he is in an automobile accident, is injured, and ends up being admitted to the orthopedic unit of a large medical-surgical hospital. Patsy arrives just as Ron is admitted and blurts out: "He was on his way to the outpatient treatment program to be treated for marijuana abuse when he had this accident. He is going to lose his job if he doesn't go for treatment. This is awful."

Questions

1. Why do you think Ron smoked the last of his marijuana before going to the first night of inpatient treatment for drug abuse? How did Ron's behavior demonstrate the difference between insight and judgment?

2. How would you respond if you were the nurse listening to the girlfriend comment about the client using marijuana before his accident and his need to complete the drug abuse treatment program in order to save his job as a teacher?

3. How would you feel if you were assigned to work with this client who has been abusing cannabis (marijuana) and teaching high school students and is now in need of medical care, possibly due to using cannabis (marijuana) then driving?

4. What are the criteria for cannabis abuse, and does this client appear to meet any of those criteria? What is the difference between someone who abuses marijuana and someone who is dependent on it?

5. Would you expect this client to have withdrawal symptoms if he does not have marijuana to smoke? How would withdrawal manifest?

6. What is/are the current treatment(s) for cannabis abuse?

7. You are to instruct Ron about harmful effects of cannabis, but he is skeptical and thinks there are no harmful effects. Has cannabis been shown to adversely affect the health of someone who abuses it?

Questions (continued)

8. Are there medical uses for cannabis, and is there a medical source or sources of cannabis?

9. Is marijuana use for medical purposes permitted in your state? If not, are there nearby states where it is?

10. Would you feel better caring for this client if he had a medical prescription for marijuana or if smoking marijuana for personal use were legal? If so, under what circumstances should a client smoke marijuana for personal use?

11. How does this client's belief in Buddhism impact or affect your care?

12. The client's mother comes to visit and you talk to her about the importance of support and compassion. She asks you to explain the difference between support and compassion and enabling. She tells you that she was told in the past not to enable Ron's abuse of marijuana.

13. If you were to write a care plan for this client, what assessment data would you like to have?

14. What nursing diagnoses would you write for this client? What goals are likely for this client?

15. What interventions would you likely write for this client?

GENDER

Female

AGE

51

SETTING

- Home/visiting nurse

ETHNICITY

- White American

CULTURAL CONSIDERATIONS

- Appalachian/Northern European descent

PREEXISTING CONDITION

- Possible Alpha-1 Antitrypsin deficiency

COEXISTING CONDITION

- Chronic Obstructive Pulmonary Disease (COPD) related to Chronic Emphysema

COMMUNICATION

DISABILITY

- Disabled due to Emphysema and COPD

SOCIOECONOMIC

- Husband on social security; client receives social security disability payments; subsidized housing

SPIRITUAL/RELIGIOUS

- Used to attend church but now too tiring to attend

PHARMACOLOGIC

- Nicotine spray
- Bupropion (Zyban)
- Ipratropium bromide (Atrovent)

PSYCHOSOCIAL

- Decreased social life due to tiring easily because of COPD and Emphysema
- External locus of control

LEGAL

- Confidentiality

ETHICAL

- Should people have the right to smoke when it harms their health and that of others in their environment?

ALTERNATIVE THERAPY

- Hypnosis
- Acupuncture
- Guided imagery

PRIORITIZATION

DELEGATION

MODERATE

NICOTINE DEPENDENCE

Level of difficulty: Moderate

Overview: Requires critical thinking to come up with strategies to motivate a client, who is disabled due to Emphysema, to give up smoking. The nurse must get the client to move beyond her external locus of control thinking. The nurse must explore her own thinking about, and issues regarding, smoking in order to be effective with the client.

Client Profile

Margaret is a 51-year-old woman who smokes a package of cigarettes a day even though she has Chronic Obstructive Pulmonary Disease (COPD) from Chronic Emphysema. She has severe shortness of breath at times during the day. She cannot walk from the car to the house or carry her own groceries without tiring. Margaret's husband, John, smokes too, but just a cigar each day in the evening along with a glass of beer. Margaret has a "little glass of beer" with him. Margaret's daughter won't let her children go to Margaret's home because of the secondhand smoke and Margaret does not have the energy to climb the stairs to her daughter's home, so she has not seen her grandchildren for over a year. John does all the cooking, and the daughter takes Margaret's list and does the shopping. Margaret does not go to the church she has attended since she was a child because she does not want her many friends there to see her so short of breath and easily exhausted.

Sometimes Margaret cuts back on the groceries she puts on her list so she can have enough money for cigarettes and beer. Her daughter won't buy the cigarettes when she does the shopping, so Margaret calls the liquor store to deliver them along with a case of beer.

Margaret developed pneumonia recently and was hospitalized for treatment. The doctor mentioned to her on discharge that it would be a good idea for her to stop smoking and that he was sending the visiting nurse to work with her to quit smoking.

Case Study

The visiting nurse calls Margaret and tells her that the doctor has asked her to stop by for a visit. Margaret says she is doing OK and doesn't think she needs to see the nurse. The nurse replies: "I'd like to see you even though you are doing fine. Would you like me to come on Tuesday at 10 AM or Thursday at 4 PM?" Margaret agrees to the Tuesday visit. When the nurse arrives at Margaret and John's home, she visits a few minutes with Margaret and John and then checks Margaret's vital signs, listens to her lungs and heart sounds, does oxygen saturation, and draws some blood to send to the lab for CBC. She checks the capillary refill and then asks Margaret if they could have a cup of tea and just visit.

The nurse has brought some "special" tea bags. The nurse makes the tea and begins to discuss smoking with Margaret. The nurse asks Margaret how long she has been smoking, and the answer is: "Since I was 18 years old." The nurse asks her if she has ever thought about quitting, and she says: "No, I need it to calm my nerves." The nurse replies: "Perhaps the doctor can prescribe something to help you calm your nerves. While there are pros to smoking like increased alertness and relaxation, there are some cons to smoking like it increases the risk of serious illness and it makes your Emphysema worse." Margaret tells the nurse that she has known lots of people who smoked and none of them got Emphysema or pulmonary disease or cancer or lung problems: "It is just bad luck that I got this Emphysema, and I have hospital insurance and cancer insurance." Margaret tells the nurse that her father raised tobacco and tobacco is a good plant. She describes how she used to help her father by cutting the blooms out of the tobacco to keep them from sucking energy from the plant. Then Margaret asks: "Do you smoke or did you ever smoke, nurse?"

Before the visit ends, the nurse asks Margaret about her ancestry. Margaret says her father's parents came from Denmark and her mother's great-grandparents came from Finland. When the nurse reports back to Margaret's doctor, she tells him that it will be difficult to get Margaret to quit smoking but that she has some ideas, and she asks him about the possibility of Alpha-1 Antitrypsin (AT) deficiency.

Questions

1. Why do you think the health care provider wants Margaret to give up smoking? What would be some common feelings of nurses assigned to work with a client like Margaret?

2. If you were the nurse, how would you respond when the client asks if you smoke or ever smoked? Do you think a nurse who smokes can help a client successfully give up smoking?

3. Margaret's family asks: "What is Emphysema and what causes it?" How would you answer? What do you know about Alpha-1 AT deficiency as a cause of Emphysema, and what clues point to the possibility Margaret could have this deficiency?

4. Why would this client, or any client, refuse to have testing for Alpha-1 AT deficiency? Why would a client want to have the testing? What are the current treatments for Alpha-1 AT deficiency and for Emphysema?

5. What are the criteria for a diagnosis of nicotine dependence, and does Margaret appear to meet these criteria? Is there a measuring tool that measures the degree of nicotine dependency of clients?

6. What are the current theories on causation of nicotine dependence?

7. What are the current treatments for nicotine dependence? Would it be easy or difficult to get someone who is nicotine dependent to give up smoking, and what would help a person who doesn't want to give up smoking?

8. Is smoking more common among lower socio-economic groups or other groups? What general characteristics of individuals from Appalachia have been identified that might be helpful to keep in mind in designing interventions to help the client stop smoking?

9. What will you do to help this client maintain a nonsmoking status if she agrees to stop smoking? How will you feel and what attitude will you adopt if she relapses again?

10. What are the withdrawal symptoms this client will probably have?

11. What data do you want to gather on this client? What nursing diagnoses, goals, and interventions would you likely write if you were writing a care plan for this client?

Bennie

GENDER	**SOCIOECONOMIC**
Male	■ Middle class
AGE	**SPIRITUAL/RELIGIOUS**
19	
SETTING	**PHARMACOLOGIC**
■ Workplace, office of industrial nurse	
ETHNICITY	**PSYCHOSOCIAL**
■ White American	
CULTURAL CONSIDERATIONS	**LEGAL**
■ American "Rave" culture	■ Illegal drug use
PREEXISTING CONDITION	**ETHICAL**
	■ Professional vs. personal relationship with client
COEXISTING CONDITION	**ALTERNATIVE THERAPY**
COMMUNICATION	**PRIORITIZATION**
DISABILITY	**DELEGATION**

HALLUCINOGEN ABUSE

Level of difficulty: High

Overview: Requires the nurse to accept a young adult whose behavior is risky to his health and who is using the illegal stimulant/hallucinogen MDMA (Ecstasy) and has a lifestyle totally different from that of the nurse. The nurse must maintain professional behavior and help the client develop a trusting relationship before attempting to motivate a change in behavior in the client.

DIFFICULT

Client Profile

Bennie is a 19-year-old adopted male, who has worn leather and chains at times in the past couple of years. His hair has occasionally been spiked up the middle of his head and colored green. His behavior has attracted attention in his parents' conservative upper-middle-class neighborhood. In addition to his hairstyle he has stood in the middle of the street and cursed his adoptive parents, talked to neighbors about smoking "weed," and played his drums loudly. The parents have been concerned about his effect on a younger brother who is their natural child and involved in sports and not at all like their adopted son. Just before graduation from high school, the parents suggested Bennie move out. Bennie moved to an apartment with one of his friends, got a job designing computer games, and started going to raves. His passions are: raves, the drug MDMA (Ecstasy), Macintosh computers, computer games, and cars. His parents have asked him not to come home.

Case Study

Bennie comes to the nurse's office in the company where he works. His chief complaints are insomnia, feeling anxious and nauseated, and experiencing blurred vision. He wants his blood pressure checked to see if something is wrong. As the nurse takes his vital signs, the nurse finds Bennie has a rapid pulse of 124 and tremors in his hands. The nurse notices that his muscles are tense and he is sweating. His mood appears a little depressed, and he thinks people in his department are sabotaging his work.

Bennie tells the nurse he thinks she is cute and asks her to go out with him. The nurse's response is: "When you go out, Bennie, where do you like to go?" The client reveals he likes to go to raves and invites the nurse to go with him to a rave.

Questions

1. If you were the female nurse in this case, would it be acceptable for you to go out socially with this client? Why or why not? What developmental stage, according to Erickson, is this client in and how does that relate to the client's behavior? Could the nurse have professional reason(s) for asking Bennie what he really likes to do in his time away from work?

2. What does the client mean by a "rave"?

3. What is the most common drug used at raves and why? What other drugs are commonly found at raves? Is there drug paraphernalia associated with MDMA (Ecstasy)? Is the typical way of dressing at raves leather and chains, and if not, what is it?

4. What drugs are considered hallucinogens? How are hallucinogens usually taken, and how is Ecstasy taken? Have there been or are there currently any medical uses for hallucinogens?

5. What effect does MDMA have on the person taking it? Is the strength of the drug MDMA consistent, and what is the danger of receiving PMA (paramethoxyamphetamine) as a substitute for MDMA?

6. Does admitting attendance at raves affirm that the client does hallucinogenic drugs? The client

admits taking MDMA. What action(s) do you take? What is your top priority with this client?

7. What are the criteria for Hallucinogen Intoxication? Does this client appear to meet those criteria?

8. What are the criteria for Hallucinogen Abuse, and does this client seem to meet the criteria for Hallucinogen Abuse? What diagnoses are associated with hallucinogens that are not associated with some other addictions such as alcohol, and what significance does this have for the nurse?

9. Has the use of Ecstasy increased or decreased in recent years? How is the prevalence of hallucinogen use, particularly that of Ecstasy, estimated?

10. What treatments are currently being used for clients who use or abuse Ecstasy?

11. What data would you like to have if you were the nurse writing a nursing care plan for this client? What nursing diagnoses and goals would you likely write for this client? What interventions could you write for this client?

12. What research is being conducted with hallucinogens?

GENDER

Female

AGE

13

SETTING

- School nurse called to the girl's restroom

ETHNICITY

- White American

CULTURAL CONSIDERATIONS

PREEXISTING CONDITION

- Neglect; physical, sexual, and psychological abuse

COEXISTING CONDITION

COMMUNICATION

DISABILITY

SOCIOECONOMIC

- Lower socioeconomic group; living below poverty line

SPIRITUAL/RELIGIOUS

PHARMACOLOGIC

PSYCHOSOCIAL

LEGAL

- Laws requiring reporting suspected child abuse
- Legal issues when child is truant

ETHICAL

- Question of when it is all right to plant an idea in the client's mind and when it is not

ALTERNATIVE THERAPY

PRIORITIZATION

- Nurse has several students needing care

DELEGATION

- Question of what to delegate to nonnursing personnel

INHALANT ABUSE

Level of difficulty: High

Overview: Requires perseverance and patience to work with a teenager who has been "huffing" gasoline and inhaling spray paint fumes. The nurse must use therapeutic communication skills, observational skills, and other means to discover what is going on with the client. The nurse is required to prioritize and delegate some tasks to others as there are other students seeking services at the same time this client is experiencing problems.

DIFFICULT

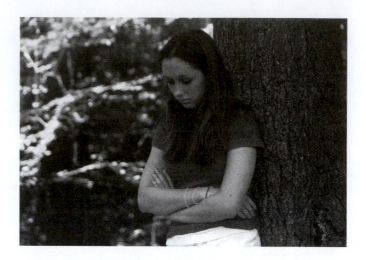

Client Profile

Pena is a 13-year-old girl whose parents are alcoholics. The family is below the poverty level in income and lives on social security disability and the food stamp program. They often sell or trade food they get with food stamps or from the WIC program to get alcohol and cigarettes, since food stamps are not accepted in payment for these items. The father tells Pena that she will never amount to anything and frequently tells her she is "stupid." Her parents don't like to ruin a good alcoholic "buzz" by eating, and they rarely prepare a meal for Pena. She eats whatever she can find in the refrigerator or cupboard. Her mother slaps Pena and yells at her. Her father sexually abuses her. Pena has learned to be as invisible as possible at home and school. She has begun to realize that some of her classmates make fun of her because she doesn't have clothes and shoes like they do and she always looks forlorn. Pena sometimes feels sorry that she is alive.

One of the neighborhood boys tells Pena she will feel better if she breathes some gasoline in a plastic bag. She has a supply of gasoline as her father keeps gasoline in a storage shed for an old lawn mower that he makes Pena use to mow the grass and weeds. She feels great for a short while after "bagging" gasoline fumes, then the old hopeless and worthless feelings return.

One day before school, after "bagging" gasoline, the boy who told her about the gasoline says he has something else they can use to feel better and gives her something else to breathe. He also touches her in some private places. Pena thinks about saying "no," but she does not care. She begins to feel euphoric. When she comes down from the high, she feels awful but goes to school because it is better than going home and she doesn't want the truancy officer visiting her home again. She hates to go to school because she can't concentrate and has little idea of what is going on in class. She is failing in school. Pena feels guilty about letting the boy touch her in private places, but he is the only one who talks to her and he has introduced her to inhalants that make her feel good, even if the feeling lasts only a short while.

Case Study

Pena passes out in the girl's bathroom at school. One of her classmates goes to get the school nurse. Pena has regained consciousness when the school nurse arrives. The nurse smells a chemical odor to Pena's breath. She seems lethargic, her movements are uncoordinated, her eyes are red, and her speech is slurred; however,

Pena does begin to respond to questions. The nurse says: "Tell me what happened." Pena replies: "I just passed out because I forgot to eat supper last night and I got up late and didn't have time for breakfast this morning." The nurse notices some gold paint on Pena's face and hands.

A student comes into the bathroom with a nosebleed, and another girl says she has just started her first menstrual period and needs a pad. It is nearly time for the nurse to begin teaching a health care class, and the truancy officer has sent word that he wants to talk to the nurse before he goes out to visit one of the families.

Questions

1. If you were the school nurse, would you say: "Tell me what happened"? Why or why not? What else would you say or do or avoid saying and/or doing when approaching this client initially? Based on the client's symptoms, what problem(s) could this client have instead of inhalant use? What are some clues that this student has been using inhalants?

2. What are the criteria for Inhalant Intoxication, and could Pena likely meet those criteria? What are the criteria for Inhalant Abuse, and does this client appear to meet any of those criteria?

3. You learn from one of Pena's classmates that several students are inhaling solvents. What are solvents? Are there different categories of inhalants that this client could have used? How are nitrites different from the other three types of solvents? Give some examples of nitrites. How are solvents used?

4. Two students (one with nosebleed and one starting a first menstrual period), the truancy officer, and a class that the nurse needs to teach compete with this client's needs for the nurse's attention. How would you prioritize and proceed, that is, what would you put on hold and/or delegate? Would you accompany Pena to the hospital if you were the nurse in this case?

5. Is it possible for the hospital emergency room staff to run a routine drug screen for inhalants on this or any client (i.e., does an inhalant like gasoline appear in the urine or blood)?

6. The client receives care at the hospital and returns to school. You ask the client to stop by your office each day and check in with you. You try to discuss the harmful effects of solvent inhalation. The client says: "I don't care." Is this a typical response from inhalant users? What are the harmful effects of solvent inhalation that you would like to discuss with Pena?

7. If you were provided training and assigned by the principal to do a support group for this client and other children who are having problems, what would be the expected benefits of this group?

8. Would you put together a homogenous or a heterogeneous support group for children? What circumstances would warrant breaking confidentiality, and who could receive the information? How would you prepare the students to know about and accept the situations that could not be kept within the group?

9. If you were the school nurse, would you educate children in the classroom about Inhalant Abuse and the dangers of using inhalants? What are the signs and symptoms you could teach parents to look for that would indicate their child might be inhaling solvents?

10. Would you expect this client to have withdrawal symptoms if she stops using inhalants? If so, what symptoms would you expect?

11. What are the current treatment(s) for Inhalant Intoxication and for Inhalant Abuse?

12. In writing a care plan for this client, what assessment data would you gather? What nursing diagnoses, goals, and interventions would you write for this client and share with the team mentioned above?

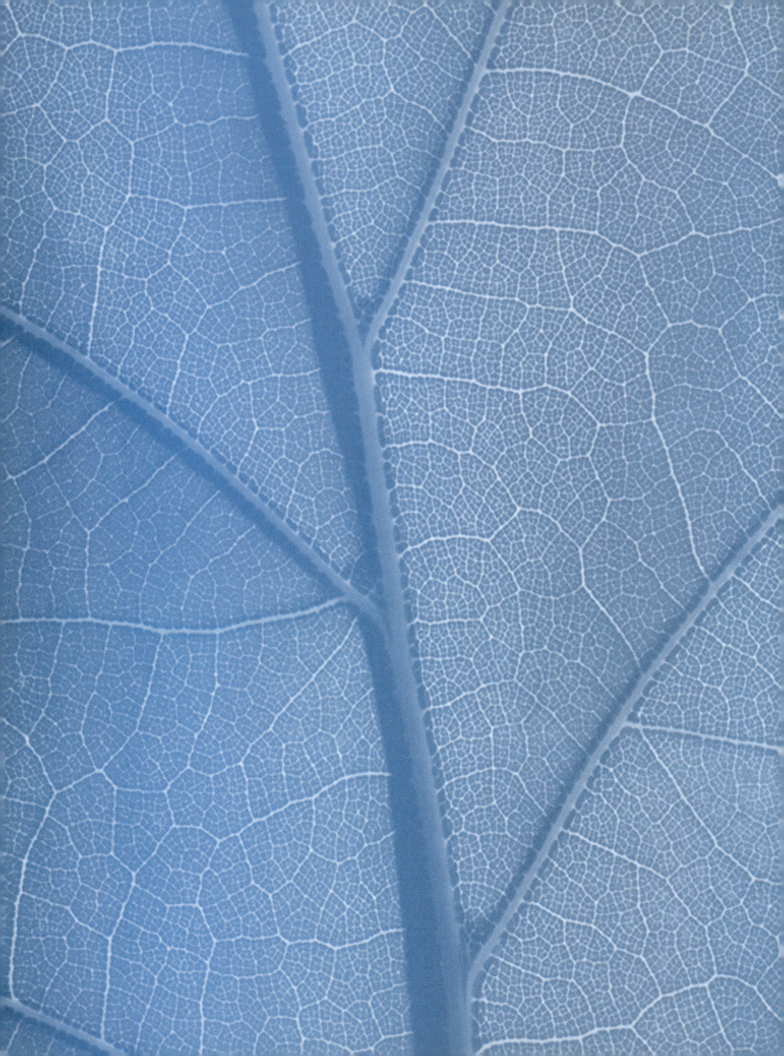

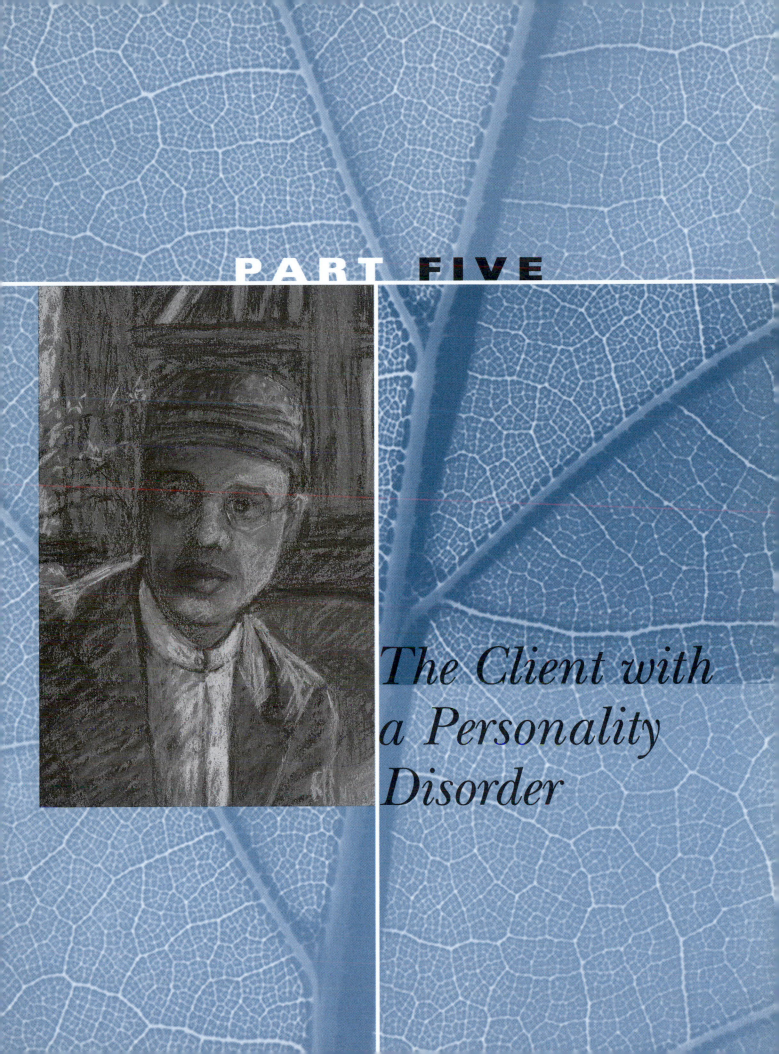

PART FIVE

The Client with a Personality Disorder

CASE STUDY 1

Vicky

GENDER

Female

AGE

27

SETTING

■ Company nurse's office

ETHNICITY

■ White American

CULTURAL CONSIDERATIONS

■ Midwestern farming culture; pioneer and Germanic influence

PREEXISTING CONDITION

COEXISTING CONDITION

COMMUNICATION

DISABILITY

SOCIOECONOMIC

■ Upper-class professional

SPIRITUAL/RELIGIOUS

PHARMACOLOGIC

PSYCHOSOCIAL

■ Desire for approval from father
■ Perfectionism and control issues interfere with social relationships

LEGAL

ETHICAL

■ Recommending one therapist: therapeutic or unethical?

ALTERNATIVE THERAPY

PRIORITIZATION

DELEGATION

OBSESSIVE-COMPULSIVE PERSONALITY DISORDER

Level of difficulty: Easy

Overview: Requires the nurse to use critical thinking to identify and understand the behavioral traits of Obsessive-Compulsive Personality Disorder (OCPD) and to determine effective therapeutic approaches. The nurse must differentiate OCPD from Obsessive-Compulsive Disorder. Requires the nurse to identify the role of the industrial nurse and to make decisions within that role.

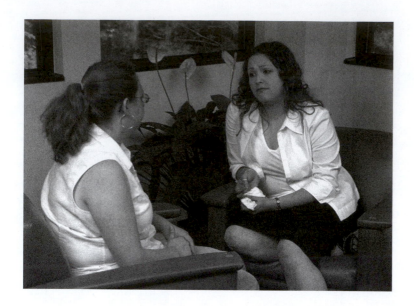

Client Profile

Vicky is a 27-year-old single woman who lives alone and works for a technology company. Vicky grew up on a midwestern small farm with frugal parents. An authoritarian father rarely said much to her except to criticize her behavior. She tried to be perfect at school, often recopying papers several times and thus failing to get them in on time, which meant only a B or C grade. Once when she got a 98 on a paper and was hopeful of getting praise at home, her father said: "What are you going to do about getting 100 next time?" By college Vicky was a straight A student, but her father still didn't praise her. Growing up, she was overly organized with everything in its place in her room and lists posted everywhere. Vicky resisted going to bed until work on the lists was done or she was exhausted and gave up. In the past few years, Vicky has had trouble getting rid of things. She tries to set things aside for charity, but eventually takes things out, one by one, and puts them back inside the house, thinking maybe she will use them some day. Although she is wealthy, she is frugal with her money.

Vicky spends hours trying to get projects at work perfect. When assigned to a project with a coworker, she does most or all of the work herself, because she thinks coworkers won't do it correctly. Sometimes she realizes coworkers are having fun on the weekend while she has no time for leisure activities. Once in awhile she misses a project deadline due to trying to perfect the work.

A former coworker and friend with a romantic interest in Vicky has repeatedly invited her to visit him in another city. Finally, Vicky accepts since she will have her own room and a housekeeper will be there. The friend takes her to a museum to see a European art collection on loan. Vicky insists on viewing the paintings starting at the entrance and going right to left, seeing each painting, reading each plaque, and making a note about it. By the time the museum closes, they have not gotten close to the collection they came to see. Before going out to eat, Vicky insists her friend change his shirt to match his pants and then change his tie. She organizes his ties by color and after some indecision selects one. Before Vicky leaves, her friend tells her he cares for her and gently asks her to see a therapist about her perfectionism and need to control.

Case Study

On Monday afternoon, Vicky presents in the nurse's office of the company where she works asking the nurse to take her blood pressure and complaining of feeling dizzy. The nurse notices that Vicky has rearranged the magazines in the office waiting area and has brought a large stack of what looks like work with her. The nurse asks her about the stack of papers. Vicky says she is behind schedule since she was out of town over the weekend. She shares that she thought maybe she would have time to do some work while waiting to see the nurse. Vicky's blood pressure is within normal limits, as are the rest of the vital signs. The nurse observes that the client looks thin and seems anxious. When the nurse assesses Vicky's heath practices and asks about diet, Vicky says: "Oh, I eat well, but sometimes I skip lunch to get some work done or I forget to eat breakfast when I get busy doing work before I come to work." She admits to getting four to five hours of sleep nightly. The nurse asks Vicky about turning some of this work over to her team members and going home to rest. Vicky seems anxious and even angry as she replies: "No one else can get it right." Then she bursts into tears and says: "A friend of mine says I am a perfectionist and controlling and I should get some help. He doesn't really understand. Do you think I should see a therapist? I really don't have time."

Questions

1. If you were the nurse talking with Vicky, how would you respond to her statements about her friend's thoughts on her perfectionism, need to control, and need to see a therapist, as well as her question to you on whether she should see a therapist or not?

2. What behaviors did Vicky exhibit in the waiting room and nurse's office that might clue the nurse to assess further for behaviors matching traits of Obsessive-Compulsive Personality Disorder?

3. If you were the nurse, what other assessments would you want to do at this time?

4. What are the traits of Obsessive-Compulsive Personality? What behaviors does Vicky have that match these traits? What are the criteria for a diagnosis of OCPD by a professional qualified to make a diagnosis?

5. Obsessive-Compulsive Personality Disorder sounds a lot like Obsessive-Compulsive Disorder. Are they two different disorders or not? Discuss how OCPD and OCD are alike and how they are different.

6. Is there any difference in the reported prevalence of this disorder in males compared to females?

7. If Vicky goes to a therapist, the therapist will probably ask about her family and her experiences growing up. Does childhood family environment possibly play a role in the development of Obsessive-Compulsive Personality Disorder? Was Vicky's father's behavior possibly culturally influenced in any way?

8. Are environmental factors the accepted cause of Obsessive-Compulsive Disorder?

9. Using Erickson's psychosocial development theory, what developmental stage is this client in and how could that play a role in her wanting to modify her behavior by working with a therapist?

10. What nursing diagnoses would you write for this client?

11. What interventions do professional counselors, therapists, or psychiatric nurse clinicians use in working with clients who have traits of OCPD or a diagnosis of this disorder? What interventions would be helpful on the part of the industrial nurse in this case?

George

GENDER

Male

AGE

39

SETTING

- Outpatient community mental health center

ETHNICITY

- White American

CULTURAL CONSIDERATIONS

- Girlfriend is Hispanic

PREEXISTING CONDITION

COEXISTING CONDITION

- Chronic depressed mood, possibly dysthymia

COMMUNICATION

DISABILITY

SOCIOECONOMIC

- Slightly above minimum wage

SPIRITUAL/RELIGIOUS

PHARMACOLOGIC

- Paroxetine (Paxil)
- Trasodone (Desyrel)

PSYCHOSOCIAL

LEGAL

- Legal obligation to provide secure e-mail if e-mailing with clients

ETHICAL

ALTERNATIVE THERAPY

PRIORITIZATION

DELEGATION

AVOIDANT PERSONALITY DISORDER

Level of difficulty: Easy

Overview: Requires recognition of the basic traits associated with Avoidant Personality Disorder and critical thinking to build a professional nurse-client relationship and keep the client engaged in treatment. Helping the client to slowly increase social contact requires careful planning, effective interventions, and patience.

Client Profile

George is a 39-year-old male who lives alone. He divides his time between work and being in his bedroom on the computer. He has rarely socialized with anyone because of a fear of being criticized or rejected. Recently George quit a day job because he thought the store owner was critical of him, when in reality the store owner wanted to promote him to day manager. George felt inadequate to be a manager, fearing he would embarrass himself in the job and be criticized more. George likes his new job better because he works nights at a convenience store and does not have to interact with many people. This job is also close to a bus stop; George cannot afford a car. He has difficulty sleeping whether he is working days or nights. When he can't sleep, he works on the computer.

George had one date with Maria, whose family is from Mexico. He went to pick her up and was greeted by her extended family. He felt totally inadequate around her family and felt he was embarrassing himself and Maria, especially after Maria told him she wanted to help him shop for clothes and offered him advice on losing weight. Now he only communicates with Maria by e-mail or telephone, telling her he is "resting up for work" or "busy" when she asks him to go somewhere with her. He fantasizes about relationships with Maria and with women he meets in chat rooms, but he does not meet with them except on the computer.

Members of George's own family criticize each other in a teasing but emotionally hurtful sort of way. He has always felt rejected and criticized by his family, but once or twice a year on special occasions, he attends a family gathering at the urging of his mother. George's father talked him into going to college, but George skipped many of the classes. His father thinks he is just a few hours short of a degree when in reality he has few credits.

Case Study

George comes to the community outpatient mental health center clinic saying his father asked him to see about an antidepressant because he is overweight and seems depressed. The nurse notices that George seems very shy, as evidenced by looking down, speaking softly, and blushing at times.

George is assessed for depression, and the nurse takes an extensive health history. George describes symptoms of a depressed mood nearly every day for several years with no episodes of deep depression or elevated mood. At one point, during the history taking, George says: "You seem busy today; perhaps I could come back another day." The nurse's reply is effective as George stays for the rest of the appointment.

During assessment, the nurse uncovers much of the information in the client profile above and does a complete review of systems and asks about past and current health problems. A head-to-toe physical assessment is postponed until the next visit. The nurse finds that in addition to being somewhat depressed in mood most of the time, George has some traits of Avoidant Personality Disorder. The nurse wonders if George has sufficient traits for a diagnosis of avoidant personality disorder

The nurse suspects that George could benefit from an antidepressant and consults with the community mental health center psychiatrist, who also talks with George and prescribes a two-week supply of samples of paroxetine (Paxil) and trasodone (Desyrel). The nurse does some education with George about the medications and gives George an appointment in two weeks' time. George responds: "My job keeps me pretty busy. I don't have much time off. Could I just e-mail and tell you how I am doing? You could mail the medication to me."

Questions

1. Discuss possible reasons for George saying to the nurse: "You seem busy today; perhaps I could come back another day." What would be a good response on the part of the nurse to this statement?

2. Why did the client receive only a two-week supply of paroxetine and trasodone instead of a month or three months supply?

3. Describe an acceptable response to George's suggestion that he could e-mail rather than keep a follow-up appointment.

4. What do you think was the rationale for delaying a head-to-toe physical assessment? Discuss the value of doing the physical examination versus delaying it.

5. The nurse observed some client behaviors that suggest this client might have Avoidant Personality Disorder. What traits does George have that match this disorder? What percentage of clients in the outpatient mental health clinic would likely meet the criteria for a diagnosis of Avoidant Personality Disorder?

6. What approach or approaches by the nurse would most likely work best with this client?

7. What cause(s) of Avoidant Personality Disorder?

8. Will paroxetine and/or trasodone change the traits of Avoidant Personality Disorder as well as the symptoms of depression?

9. What education does the nurse need to do with George in regard to paroxetine (Paxil)?

10. What is the most likely reason that this client stopped seeing Maria, the girl he once dated and now only e-mails? Would her Hispanic culture present any special challenges/problems in a relationship with George and his Avoidant Personality Disorder traits?

11. What treatment(s) has been found to be helpful to the client with Avoidant Personality Disorder?

12. What nursing diagnoses would you write for this client? What goals would you likely write in collaboration with the client? Describe one or more interventions and identify how you would apply the evaluation part of nursing process.

GENDER

Male

AGE

55

SETTING

■ Client's home

ETHNICITY

■ White American

CULTURAL CONSIDERATIONS

■ Military culture
■ Wife is Japanese

PREEXISTING CONDITION

COEXISTING CONDITION

■ Chronic back pain
■ Diabetes Type II

COMMUNICATION

DISABILITY

SOCIOECONOMIC

■ Middle class: retired military and disability pay; wife has no income

SPIRITUAL/RELIGIOUS

PHARMACOLOGIC

PSYCHOSOCIAL

■ Death of mother

LEGAL

■ Confidentiality

ETHICAL

ALTERNATIVE THERAPY

■ Massage; chiropractic treatments

PRIORITIZATION

DELEGATION

DEPENDENT PERSONALITY DISORDER

Level of difficulty: Easy

Overview: Requires identification of effective ways to work with an individual who not only has traits of Dependent Personality Disorder, but also has chronic pain. Requires critical thinking to determine what culturally influenced behaviors of the spouse are enabling the husband's dependence and how to work with the spouse to modify her behavior.

Client Profile

Jim is a 55-year-old male who has both psychological and medical problems. He sees a nurse psychotherapist, goes to a pain clinic, a massage therapist, and a chiropractor for help with what he describes as uncontrollable back pain; he sees an internist for his diabetes; and he has a visiting nurse working with both him and his wife with a goal of increasing his independence in activities of daily living, exercises, and diabetes control.

In individual therapy Jim reveals a nanny cared for him for six months when he was separated from his mother at age two, due to his mother's hospitalization for treatment of major depression. Jim's father was overly protective as Jim was adopted and his father feared social services would find a reason to take Jim away. When Jim's mother returned home, Jim felt anxious when away from her.

Jim married young and joined the army. He turned every responsibility he could over to his wife whether he was home on leave or away on duty. Shortly before he retired from the army, his wife "burned out" from doing so much for him and left him for another man who paid attention to her needs. Jim immediately married Mari, a Japanese woman who seemed willing to take care of him. He then separated from the army with retirement and disability pay for a back injury. Jim's mother died two years ago, and he is still depressed about her death. He fears his wife and caregivers will reject him because he is not worthy of their attention. Jim's wife wants to go to Japan to visit her family, but when she mentions it, Jim becomes "clingy." Jim says he can't make a trip due to his bad back, which gets worse when Mari mentions a trip. Jim won't let her go, fearing something will happen to her and he'll have no one to care for him.

Case Study

The visiting nurse arrives at the client's home. Earlier in the day, the client's wife had called the nurse and described Jim becoming dizzy while shopping with her. She shared that she is now pushing Jim in a wheelchair. She stated she could do the shopping alone, but her husband insists on going with her. She said Jim often becomes angry with clerks in the stores and berates them, and this embarrasses

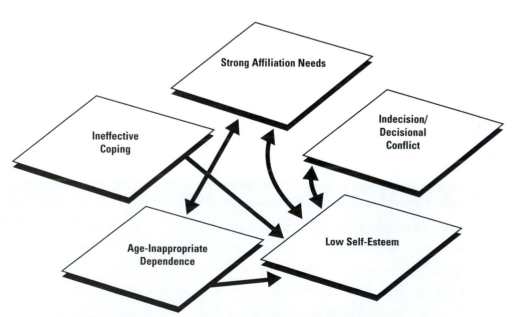

Concept map of issues and problems associated with Dependent Personality Disorder

her. She thinks he is on too much pain medication and it is causing him to be forgetful and dizzy at times. Mari said that Jim won't make decisions, has her pick out his clothes for the day, and won't do any tasks on his own initiative. She has to remind him to do his blood sugar testing and then he wants her to do it. Before the conversation ended, Mari added: "Jim needs constant care. I am getting tired. I am worried that he will get worse."

Jim greets the visiting nurse and says he needs help deciding what to do about his back pain. It is not getting better, and he has to take more pain medication and anti-anxiety medication. He can't do the exercises the doctor prescribed because it hurts too much; maybe if she would give him a massage and help him exercise, he could do a little exercise. He asks the nurse: "Would you also check my blood sugar before you do the massage?" The nurse recalls that Jim has been taught to check his own blood sugar.

Questions

1. Why would the visiting nurse need to discuss this client's case with his other care providers as well as Jim and his wife? Does the nurse need to get a release of information signed by the client before discussing his case?

2. What is a person with Dependent Personality Disorder like?

3. If you were the visiting nurse and had all the information available about Jim from other health care providers, as well as your own observations, what traits of Dependent Personality Disorder would you identify in this client?

4. What causes Dependent Personality Disorder?

5. What would be a helpful response on the part of the visiting nurse when Jim asks her to check his blood sugar?

6. What nursing diagnoses would you write for Jim if you were the visiting nurse?

7. The visiting nurse and others caring for the client, including the spouse, are scheduled to meet for a planning conference. What goals or outcomes do you think the team might come up with? Should Jim meet with the team?

8. Would Mari's cultural background have an impact on how she relates to Jim's dependency needs? How would you work with her in terms of culturally generated behavioral tendencies?

9. What general approaches do you think might be helpful for the nurse to use in working with Jim or any other client with Dependent Personality Disorder? What types of treatment modalities have been found to be helpful in working with clients with Dependent Personality Disorder?

10. What interventions would you write and utilize in regard to one or more of this client's nursing diagnoses?

11. Is Dependent Personality Disorder common in clients with medical disorders in general and with chronic pain specifically?

12. Do clients with Dependent Personality Disorder seek treatment, and if so, under what conditions?

Brad

GENDER

Male

AGE

62

SETTING

- Private psychiatric hospital outpatient clinic

ETHNICITY

- White American

CULTURAL CONSIDERATIONS

PREEXISTING CONDITION

- High blood pressure
- High cholesterol

COEXISTING CONDITION

COMMUNICATION

DISABILITY

SOCIOECONOMIC

- Affluent
- Professional

SPIRITUAL/RELIGIOUS

- Attends a church with prestigious upper-class members

PHARMACOLOGIC

PSYCHOSOCIAL

- Seeks relationships with people viewed as special or important

LEGAL

- Keeping information provided by a spouse confidential from the other spouse

ETHICAL

ALTERNATIVE THERAPY

- Chiropractic
- Massage therapy
- Health club workouts with trainer

PRIORITIZATION

- Needs of client with Narcissistic Personality Disorder vs. needs of partner

DELEGATION

MODERATE

NARCISSISTIC PERSONALITY DISORDER

Level of difficulty: Moderate

Overview: Requires knowledge of Narcissistic Personality Disorder and the use of therapeutic communication skills to work with the client. The nurse will need to help the client identify the needs he has to meet for himself and those that cause distress in his relationships.

Client Profile

Brad is a 62-year-old married male whose recall of growing up includes a feeling of feast or famine in terms of attention or lack of attention by his mother. She either smothered him with too much attention or was too busy to give him any attention. His father's business was also unpredictable, resulting in the family having lots of money most of the time with occasional periods of having to move to less pretentious housing or change from private school to public school for a semester or two, both traumatic events to a young boy. When Brad started high school, he was back in private school and his father had bought a boat. Having a boat made Brad popular with the girls, and he learned the importance of having special possessions that would attract desirable people into his company and make him feel important. He went to law school and became a lawyer. He studied finance and became a stockbroker and later began managing large financial portfolios. All these activities helped lessen his fear of losing special status and brought him into contact with prestigious people.

Brad married Mary, a girl with money and family prestige. After many years, Mary has developed health problems and is concerned that Brad had no empathy for her health situation. She is irritated at Brad frequently asking her to drop whatever she is doing and meet him somewhere or do something for him. She suspects he has had a number of affairs. After a trip to a local prestigious private psychiatric outpatient clinic, Mary tells Brad she expects him to get therapy at the clinic or she may divorce him.

Case Study

On hearing from Mary that she has been to the outpatient clinic and is thinking about divorce, Brad agrees to go alone and do a preliminary intake meeting with the staff nurse. The threat of Mary leaving him, rather than him leaving her, distresses him. Brad presents himself at the outpatient clinic. He is well-dressed and well-groomed and appears somewhat arrogant and haughty in wanting to check the credentials of the staff and dropping some names of important doctors that he knows. He states that he expects to be seen on time, as time is money in his business. He wants to use the center telephone to make some important business calls even though a sign says the telephone is for staff use only. He displays a money clip with a large number of bills and flashes a large diamond ring. He gives the impression that he is someone important and is entitled to special privileges. He calls and has a large gift basket delivered to the health care provider's home.

As the staff nurse begins the intake process, she recalls that Brad's wife, Mary, described Brad as lacking empathy and consideration and probably having affairs in the past, but the nurse is determined to keep an open mind as she gathers data from Brad. The nurse notices that Brad answers questions briefly, then asks questions about the nurse's qualifications. Brad seems to know a lot about the medications he is taking for elevated blood pressure and cholesterol and tests the nurse's knowledge about these medications and seems to enjoy any time the nurse knows less than he does about the medication.

Brad manages to mention that he owns a vacation home in an exotic location. He describes important people that he has taken there and mentions he might take the nurse to his vacation home. The nurse replies: "Let's get back to the questions on the assessment" and asks about Brad's relationship with his wife. Brad paints a picture of being very generous with his wife and her being stubborn, unloving, and unappreciative. Brad does not reveal a series of affairs throughout the years or that there is a woman he fantasizes about as an ideal lover and mate. The nurse notes that Brad seems concerned that he is aging, and this seems to be a major stressor for him. He reveals he is spending time and money seeing chiropractors and massage therapists and working out in the most prestigious health club in town. At the end of the session, the nurse suspects Brad meets a number of the criteria for Narcissistic Personality Disorder. Before Brad leaves, he says to the nurse: "I would love to know what my wife told you about me." The nurse will present the intake information to the team, and a therapist or therapists will be assigned to Brad and his wife, Mary.

Questions

1. When the nurse hears Brad say he might take her to his vacation home, she replies: "Let's get back to the questions on the assessment." What technique is she using, and what is a rationale for this reply? What is a likely rationale for Brad suggesting the trip to the nurse and for sending the health care provider a large gift basket?

2. What are the criteria for a diagnosis of Narcissistic Personality Disorder (NPD), and which criteria does Brad seem to meet?

3. Most persons with a diagnosis of Narcissistic Personality Disorder are of what gender? How often are persons diagnosed with Narcissistic Personality Disorder hospitalized specifically for treatment of this disorder?

4. Describe Kohut's and/or Kernberg's theory of causation of Narcissistic Personality Disorder.

5. What possible motivation is behind Brad calling Mary to meet him at a moment's notice? How would you feel and what would you need if you were Mary?

6. What would it feel like to be Brad? How would Brad and others with NPD likely react to changes associated with aging?

7. What will the nurse therapist most likely need to do to keep Brad engaged in couples therapy? Would there be any advantages to the nurse therapist bringing in a second therapist or cotherapist to work with this couple? What does Brad need to gain from therapy?

8. What will the therapist most likely need to do to help Mary get her needs met in this relationship?

9. How does the staff nurse need to respond to Brad's statement: "I would love to know what my wife told you about me"?

10. If you were a nurse in a health care provider's office or on a medical unit in the hospital and your assessment of a client revealed some narcissistic personality traits, would you plan your care differently to work more effectively with this client, and if so, how?

Leah

GENDER

Female

AGE

22

SETTING

- University health center

ETHNICITY

- White American

CULTURAL CONSIDERATIONS

- Sorority house culture

PRE-EXISTING CONDITION

CO-EXISTING CONDITION

COMMUNICATION

DISABILITY

SOCIOECONOMIC

- Affluent

SPIRITUAL/RELIGIOUS

PHARMACOLOGIC

PSYCHOSOCIAL

LEGAL

- Providing female nurse presence during physical examination of female client by male health care provider to avoid a false claim of sexual misconduct.

ETHICAL

- Protecting female client from misconduct by male physician during physical examination.

ALTERNATIVE THERAPY

PRIORITIZATION

- Nurse decision to accept phone call versus remaining present during physical examination.

DELEGATION

- Male nurse delegates assisting male health care provider with physical exam to female nurse peer.

Level of difficulty: Easy

Overview: Requires understanding of Histrionic Personality Disorder (HPD). Requires critical thinking to avoid legal ramifications for the professional staff, especially for the male health care provider and male nurse. The nurse must also identify effective techniques for working with the client with HPD.

Client Profile

Leah is a 22-year-old female college student who has always seemed to be the center of attention in her family, in school, and in her peer group. Although Leah's sister has many material things from their affluent family, she can't seem to get any attention from their parents. When Leah enters a room, it is with great dramatic flair. She spends a great deal of energy, time, and money on her appearance and dresses seductively. Leah has been known to fish for compliments. She is flirtatious and sometimes insinuates that she is intimate or close to important males when there is not a close relationship at all. Leah appears uncomfortable when she is not the center of attention and goes to great lengths to regain status. Leah says things like "He is such a difficult person." She gives no details and leaves the recipient of this statement wondering what she meant. Leah frequently goes through a variety of emotions rather quickly.

Case Study

Leah comes to the student health center seeking care for the "very worst cold" she has ever had. She tells the male nurse that it may be pneumonia or worse. She wonders if she should get an important close friend to fly her to Florida in his private plane. She says she feels like she will die if she does not get some sun. Later Leah mentions she might need to go to the Mayo Clinic and see the chief of the medical staff who is a close friend of her father's.

The male nurse asks the health care provider to wait a few minutes before the physical examination on Leah. He asks a female nurse peer to assist the male health care provider. The female nurse is with the health care provider when he examines Leah. The nurse thinks Leah is engaging in seductive behavior around the health care provider. Leah suggests she might need the health care provider to make a house call. Leah has obviously spent a lot of time grooming for the occasion but says to the health care provider. "I am so sick. I must look awful. Do you think I look dreadful?" The female nurse receives a message that she has an urgent telephone call, and she wonders if she can leave the examining room. The health care provider is almost finished with the examination and ready to tell Leah to get dressed.

Before Leah leaves the clinic, she dramatically approaches the male nurse saying that she is horribly depressed and maybe that is why she got a cold. Her boyfriend broke up with her and she is "just devastated." She then says: "Maybe, darling, you would be willing to make a house call to my sorority house?" The nurse responds: "I would be glad to sit and talk with you for a few minutes here at the clinic." Leah responds: "Oh well, if you don't make house calls, perhaps you would take me to the football game. I think you could make me feel much better."

Leah goes to the football game with a friend and tells the friend that "Bill" the health care provider at the clinic wanted to take her to the game, but he had to work. She suddenly yells out a girl's name and runs down the steps in the middle of the ballgame, struggles across a row of people, and hugs a girl in the middle of the row. Leah then turns to the crowd during a play that most people are trying to watch and yells out dramatically, "This is my old roommate and I haven't seen her for a month."

Questions

1. What personality trait of a person with a diagnosis of Histrionic Personality Disorder is usually most noticeable? Which of Leah's behaviors make you suspect she has this personality trait?

2. Could Leah or anyone else have personality traits of Histrionic Personality Disorder and not have the disorder itself? If yes, what behaviors would Leah have to have to get this diagnosis and does she have these behaviors?

3. Why did the male nurse delegate the task of assisting the health care provider with the physical examination to a female nurse? If you were the female nurse in the examining room with the health care provider while he examined Leah, what would you do if someone came and told you that you had an urgent telephone call? Give a rationale for your decision.

4. Did the male nurse respond appropriately when Leah suggested he make a house call? Why or why not?

5. If you were the male nurse, how would you have responded when Leah asked you to take her to the football game?

6. Based on your limited knowledge of Leah's behavior, what nursing diagnoses do you suppose would most likely apply in her case?

7. What nursing interactions might be of help to Leah?

8. What treatment interventions are currently being used in the treatment of Histrionic Personality Disorder?

9. Do clients with Histrionic Personality Disorder get better?

10. What causes Histrionic Personality Disorder?

GENDER

Male

AGE

36

SETTING

- Emergency room

ETHNICITY

- White American

CULTURAL CONSIDERATIONS

PREEXISTING CONDITION

COEXISTING CONDITION

- Fractured arm

COMMUNICATION

DISABILITY

SOCIOECONOMIC

- Low-paid, white-collar government worker with good health benefits

SPIRITUAL/RELIGIOUS

- Is not a "joiner"
- Prefers to worship alone

PHARMACOLOGIC

PSYCHOSOCIAL

LEGAL

ETHICAL

- Nurse's spouse has relationship with client
- Nurse has potential for dual relationship with client
- Strict confidentiality vs. selective breach to nurse's spouse

ALTERNATIVE THERAPY

PRIORITIZATION

DELEGATION

SCHIZOID PERSONALITY DISORDER

Level of difficulty: High

Overview: Requires critical thinking to assure confidentiality in a situation in which the nurse and the nurse's spouse each have a professional relationship with the client and the nurse has potential for a dual relationship. Requires critical thinking in determining effective means of communicating with a client who prefers to be alone and does not enjoy interacting with others.

DIFFICULT

Client Profile

Howard is a 36-year-old male who was raised by his father after his mother died when he was 6 months old. The father was absent a lot from Howard's life due to his work and dating the same woman for twenty years before he suddenly died. Howard only met the father's girlfriend a handful of times and was raised by a strict grandmother. Howard stayed away from grandmother as much as he could so he would not be punished.

As Howard grew up, he became fascinated with computers and now calls himself a computer "geek." He works in a remote office inputting computer data and doing research for a state agency. He keeps track of the milk production of cows by county throughout the state. The pay is fairly low, but he does not have to go to meetings or interface with anyone except for meeting twice each month with his supervisor. Howard's work earned an award in his state agency, but he would not go to the dinner to accept the award. His supervisor picked the award up for him.

Howard is described by others as pretty much a "loner": living alone, never trying to make friends, and never joining any group. He does not attend a church, preferring to read the bible and pray alone. A first cousin and childhood playmate of Howard recalls that Howard has stayed away from family activities ever since he was old enough not to require a babysitter. Once in awhile the cousin goes to visit him, but Howard never initiates a visit to the cousin. The cousin recalls that Howard's facial expression has always been somewhat flat, and as a child he did not mimic her when she would smile or make faces. The cousin has never noticed any behavior that would indicate Howard is interested sexually in women or perhaps men. A neighbor once tried to start a relationship, but she noticed that Howard became anxious whenever she came near him and he was somewhat cold and aloof.

Case Study

Howard has been brought to the emergency room by EMS. The emergency medical technician (EMT) reports that Howard had apparently been riding his bicycle to work when the driver of a car, claiming to have been blinded by the sun, hit him. The EMT further reports that Howard wanted to go home when he talked with the policeman on the scene, but finally agreed to come to the ER to get checked out for injuries.

When the ER receptionist asks Howard if she can call any of his family or a friend for him or if he would like to call them, he responds: "No." He hides behind a book in the corner of the ER until the x-ray technician comes to x-ray his arm, which he has said hurts and has some pins-and-needles-like feeling.

When the health care provider views the x-ray, it is clear that the ulna is broken. The provider shares with the emergency room nurse that he wants to reset the broken bone, cast the arm, and keep Howard overnight. The nurse goes to tell Howard what the provider plans to do.

After surgery, Howard is taken to his room. It is late in the evening shift when he arrives at his room. When the nurse gets her assignments and receives report, she goes to do the initial assessment on Howard and finds him wide awake. She introduces herself. Howard says: "That is an interesting and unusual last name. My supervisor at work must be related to you. His name is Mark." The night nurse realizes that Howard's supervisor is her husband and that she may see Howard in the future when she attends activities at her husband's workplace.

Questions

1. Does Howard demonstrate traits of Schizoid Personality Disorder (SZPD), and if so, what traits?

2. Can a person described as a "loner" with all or most of the traits of Schizoid Personality Disorder still not meet all the requirements for a diagnosis of SZPD? If so, what additional requirement has to be met?

3. Looking at Howard's behaviors, what makes you more certain they are those associated with SZPD and not those of Avoidant Personality Disorder?

4. If you were the female nurse going to tell Howard about the health care provider's plans to set his arm and cast it and keep him overnight, what would you keep in mind as you plan your approach? What would you say to this client, and how would you say it?

5. If you were the female nurse ready to do the initial assessment of this client and he discovered that you were the wife of his supervisor, what options would you have and which one would you select?

6. What nursing diagnoses, in addition to acute pain and impaired skin integrity for his broken arm, would you write for this client in relation to traits of SZPD?

7. How would you go about writing goals for this client, and what goals might you write if the client is to stay in the rehabilitation hospital for several days or weeks?

8. What interventions might the nurse implement?

9. What are some theories of causation of Schizoid Personality Disorder?

10. What is the current treatment for Schizoid Personality Disorder?

Stan

GENDER

Male

AGE

32

SETTING

- Outpatient mental health center clinic

ETHNICITY

- Black/White American

CULTURAL CONSIDERATIONS

- White American father, Black American mother

PREEXISTING CONDITION

COEXISTING CONDITION

- Hypertension

COMMUNICATION

DISABILITY

SOCIOECONOMIC

SPIRITUAL/RELIGIOUS

PHARMACOLOGIC

- Captopril in combination with hydrochlorthiazide (Capozide)
- Lorazepam (Ativan)
- Olanzapine (Zyprexa)

PSYCHOSOCIAL

- Paranoia limits and distorts interactions with others

LEGAL

ETHICAL

ALTERNATIVE THERAPY

- Over-the-counter vitamins, minerals, and enzymes

PRIORITIZATION

DELEGATION

PARANOID PERSONALITY DISORDER

Level of difficulty: High

Overview: Requires critical thinking and decision making in regard to who is going to be most effective in interacting with the client when the client's paranoia worsens. The nurse is required to work collaboratively with other team members and to provide supervision for the client's nonnurse case manager who works with the client in his independent living situation. The nurse is required to work with physical problems as well as mental health problems and to look at possible connections between psychological and medical problems and the medications used to treat them.

DIFFICULT

Client Profile

Stan is a 32-year-old single male. Stan lives alone in a government-subsidized apartment and receives social security disability income (SSDI). He says he stays away from his neighbors, as they are not to be trusted and could turn against him for no reason at all if he were to let them into his apartment.

Stan holds grudges against his mother and has not attempted to contact her for a couple of years. He talks about his mother trying to control his mind and his life and working against him to get him into treatment when he did not want or need it. He carries a grudge over his mother not giving him a birthday party ten years ago when his brother got a party: "Not that I wanted one, but it just was not fair of my mom to do that." Stan is also angry at his mother for giving him a White American father so Black American peers did not accept him and for her being Black American and causing him not to be accepted by White American peers when he was growing up. He was married briefly to Yvonne, a Black American woman he met in group therapy. He was extremely jealous of Yvonne talking to other people and thought she was unfaithful when he heard her talking to a "Bobby" on the phone. Bobbie was a girl his wife had met when she was an inpatient in the psychiatric hospital. This prompted him to follow his wife everywhere she went and to try to keep her home whenever he could to prevent her from meeting this "other man." Stan was verbally hostile to his wife at times, thinking she was criticizing him when in fact she was complimenting him. Stan was jealous every time Yvonne went for psychiatric treatment. He thought she was "hogging all the therapy" (i.e., getting more than her share of psychiatric care).

Stan gets psychiatric care through the county outpatient mental health center clinic. He has a nonnurse case manager who takes vital signs, supervises him in taking his daily medication, helps him with managing his money, and transports him to appointments at the clinic where he sees a psychiatric mental health nurse for all his medication reviews and health assessments. He sees the psychiatrist only if the nurse refers him, and this usually happens only if he is experiencing a significant change in his mental health, has medical problems or problems with his medications, or needs to have additional medication prescribed. Stan currently has prescriptions for two medications: a pill for hypertension (captopril [Capozide 25/15]) and a multivitamin. His medicine cabinet is full of various kinds of vitamins, minerals, and enzymes.

Case Study

Stan reports in at the reception desk at the mental health center clinic. The nurse is walking out to call him into her office about the same time he notices two women talking across the waiting room. He calls out a derogatory name and tells them to stop talking about him. When he sees the nurse, he puts his hands on his hips in a threatening kind of stance and says: "You think you are so smart, but I know what you put in those pills. Don't think you fooled me. And don't put that in my chart." The nurse feels a great deal of energy coming from Stan and feeling threatened; she senses she needs to back away from him. The nurse says gently: "Please sit down and rest for just a few minutes. I'll have your caseworker sit with you, and in a little while when you are ready to talk she can come and get me."

The nurse alerts the psychiatrist that she is going to try to talk with Stan about his medication, but that if Stan is too paranoid, she may need the psychiatrist to discuss his medications with him. The nurse knows from working with Stan for a while and reading his chart that he has a diagnosis of Paranoid Personality Disorder.

When the psychiatrist sees Stan he notes that Stan's blood pressure is still elevated and that he is paranoid and somewhat psychotic. The psychiatrist continues the Capozide and vitamin and orders lorazepam (Ativan) and olanzapine (Zyprexa).

Questions

1. How would you feel and what would you think if you were assigned to work with Stan or any client has Paranoid Personality Disorder?

2. If you were the nurse and Stan said to you: "You think you are so smart," and you felt threatened, what would you think is going on with Stan?

3. What concept or rationale did the nurse possibly have in mind when she alerted the psychiatrist that she might need to have him go over Stan's medications?

4. What behaviors does Stan have that match those of someone with Paranoid Personality Disorder?

5. Is Paranoid Personality Disorder apparent in childhood and adolescence, and if so, what behaviors would clue the family and/or clinicians that a child has this disorder?

6. Some of the behaviors that qualify a person for a diagnosis of Paranoid Personality Disorder seem similar to other personality disorders. How can a person differentiate between PPD and other personality disorders, especially Schizotypal Personality Disorder (SZPD)?

7. How does Paranoid Personality differ from Schizophrenia, Paranoid Type?

8. What is the current treatment for Paranoid Personality Disorder?

9. What does the nurse need to know about the antihypertensive, antianxiety, and antipsychotic medications the client is on? Is there any connection between the client's race and taking one or more of these medications? What do these three medications have in common?

10. What assessment would you want/need to do if you were the nurse in this case? Given the information you have on this client, what nursing diagnoses would you write?

11. What goals would you write for this client? What interventions would be helpful?

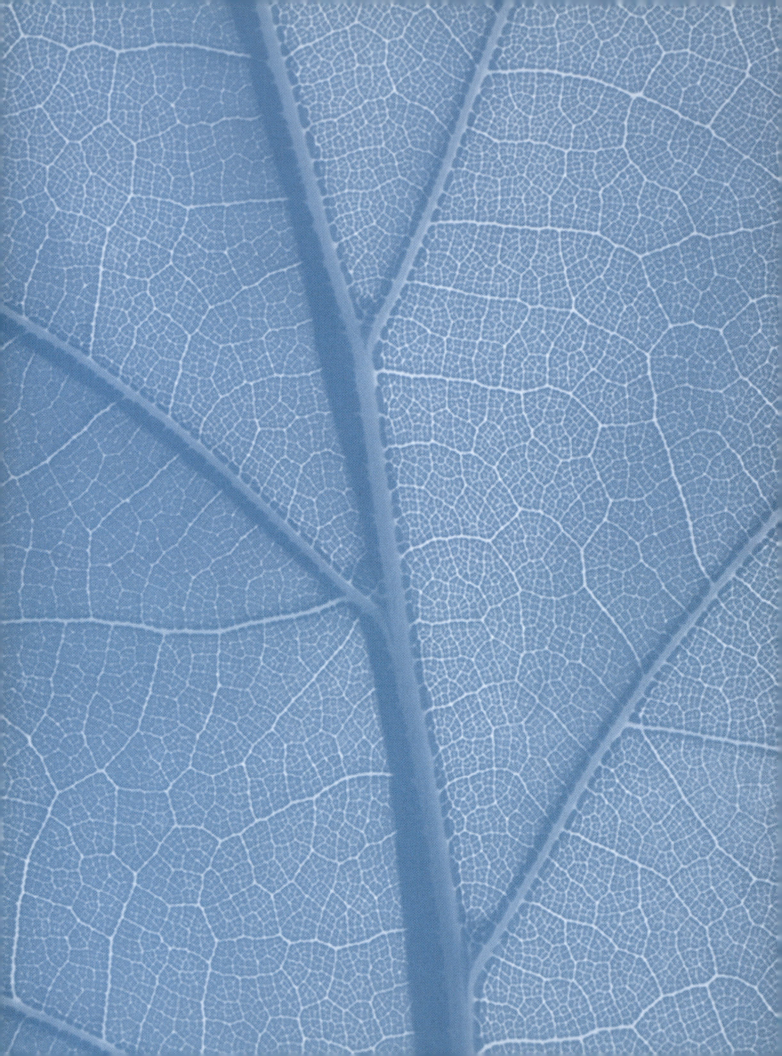

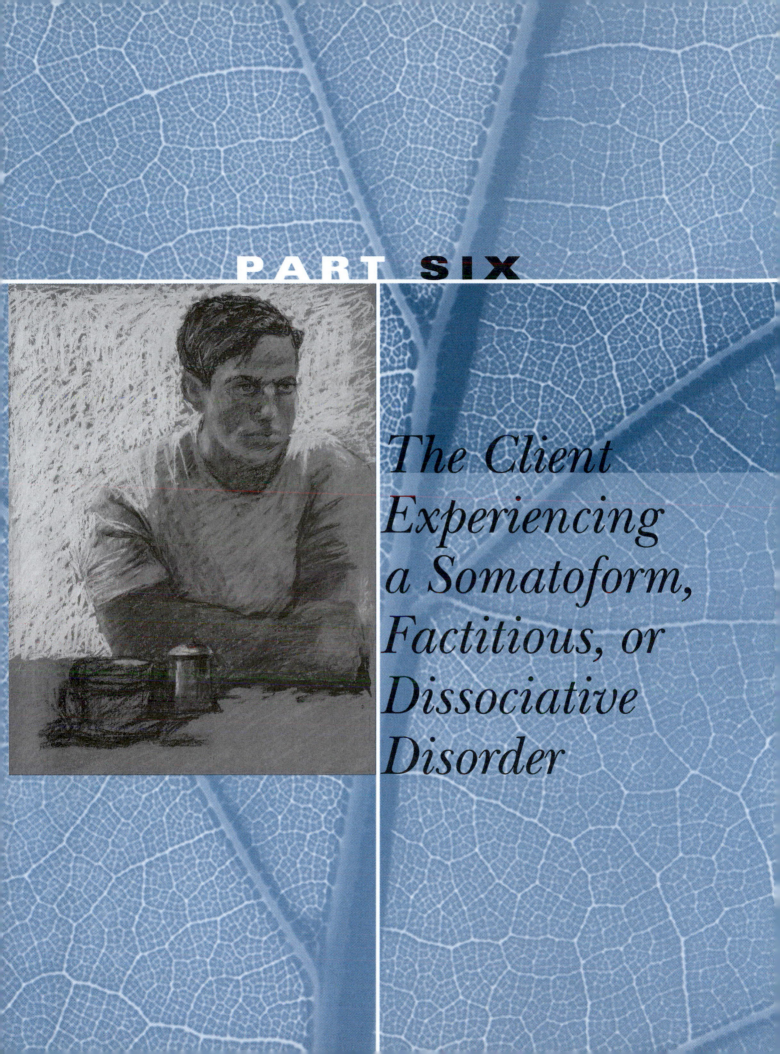

PART SIX

The Client Experiencing a Somatoform, Factitious, or Dissociative Disorder

Sarah Jane

GENDER

Female

AGE

15

SETTING

- Emergency room

ETHNICITY

- White American father and Chilean American mother

CULTURAL CONSIDERATIONS

- Germanic and Hispanic

PREEXISTING CONDITION

COEXISTING CONDITION

COMMUNICATION

DISABILITY

SOCIOECONOMIC

SPIRITUAL/RELIGIOUS

PHARMACOLOGIC

PSYCHOSOCIAL

LEGAL

- Possible lawsuit if Conversion Disorder is misdiagnosed and treated in error as a medical or neurological condition

ETHICAL

ALTERNATIVE THERAPY

PRIORITIZATION

DELEGATION

CONVERSION DISORDER

Level of difficulty: Easy

Overview: Requires realization that Conversion Disorder results from a subconscious defense mechanism and is not something within the client's control. Effective interventions will need to convey caring and empathy for the client without alienating the client's parents. Requires anyone working with the client to set aside any negative feelings or desire to confront the client.

Client Profile

Sarah Jane is a 15-year-old adolescent whose mother was born and raised in Chile and whose father's family was from Germany three generations back. She and her parents live on a small rural northern farm. She has wanted to play the piano like her paternal grandmother, but her mother has insisted she learn to play the violin. Her father, who is very authoritarian, told her: "Do as your mother asks." Now after eight years of violin lessons twice a week after school and on Saturday, Sarah Jane believes she is not very good at playing the violin. Sarah Jane practices hard to learn a lengthy and complicated piece of music for an important recital coming up. At the recital, Sarah Jane begins to play with her music teacher accompanying her on the piano. Sarah Jane looks up and sees her mother, who has seldom left the house because of agoraphobia and who has never come to a recital before, coming in late. Sarah Jane has forgotten which notes come next. She stops playing, and her teacher has her start over. Suddenly Sarah Jane realizes she cannot hold the violin up with her left hand. Her arm is paralyzed from the elbow to the fingertips.

Case Study

Sarah Jane has been taken to the emergency room in the small town hospital where she was playing her recital. The health care provider has completed a number of neurological tests, taken x-rays, and gotten an MRI. The physical assessment and vital signs were within normal limits. Sarah Jane is admitted to the hospital for observation. The primary nurse assigned to her does an admission assessment and finds it remarkable that this client does not seem concerned about her loss of the use of her left arm from the elbow to the fingertips. The doctor comes in and raises the client's paralyzed arm directly above the client's head. The client's arm remains above the head for a few seconds and then falls out to the client's side. The doctor writes in the client's chart: "Rule Out Conversion Disorder."

Questions

1. What is Conversion Disorder? What symptoms does this client have that are consistent with Conversion Disorder?

2. What are the current theories about what causes Conversion Disorder?

3. If this client had symptoms of Conversion Disorder, why did the health care provider order more tests? Why did the provider put the client's affected arm above her head and leave it unsupported?

4. Do people with Conversion Disorder deliberately produce the symptoms for secondary gain?

5. What subtypes of Conversion Disorder are there? Which subtype of Conversion Disorder does this client seem to have? Does this subtype always produce symptoms of paralysis, or could other symptoms be produced instead? If so, what symptoms?

6. Does this client's onset of symptoms fit within the general onset of Conversion Disorder? What will be this client's course if she follows a typical course associated with Conversion Disorder?

7. What stage of development, according to Erickson, is this client trying to master? What roles might stage of development and culture play in this client's development of Conversion Disorder?

8. What information in data gathering or assessing would be helpful to the treatment team as well as the nurse?

9. What nursing diagnoses would you likely write for a client with Conversion Disorder?

10. What treatment goals would you likely write for this client? What interventions do you think would likely work well with this client?

11. What treatment approaches are reported in the literature?

GENDER

Female

AGE

51

SETTING

■ Home with visiting nurse

ETHNICITY

■ African

CULTURAL CONSIDERATIONS

■ African

PREEXISTING CONDITION

COEXISTING CONDITION

COMMUNICATION

DISABILITY

SOCIOECONOMIC

SPIRITUAL/RELIGIOUS

PHARMACOLOGIC

PSYCHOSOCIAL

■ Socialization altered by client's focus on physical symptoms

LEGAL

■ Possible lawsuit for unnecessary surgery, especially if complications from surgery or if an actual medical problem occurs and is missed

ETHICAL

ALTERNATIVE THERAPY

PRIORITIZATION

DELEGATION

MODERATE

SOMATIZATION DISORDER

Level of difficulty: Moderate

Overview: Requires critical thinking and decision making about when to listen to symptoms and when to refocus the client on the task at hand. Involves critical thinking in terms of assessing and identifying problems that are current and need to be the focus of interventions.

Client Profile

Melba is a 51-year-old married female of African birth who immigrated to the United States with her parents when she was 15 years old. She has a history of numerous physical complaints and several surgeries. She is presently recuperating at home from exploratory surgery. She had complained of abdominal pain, changes in bowel habits, abdominal bloating, nausea, and vomiting, and after numerous trips to a variety of health care providers who prescribed a number of medications for the pain, nausea, and constipation, she found a surgeon who thought an exploratory laparotomy was warranted. No pathology was found during this surgery. Melba's hospital stay was extended due to an infection at the incisional site and then she was sent home on antibiotics and wet to dry dressings. On discharge, instructions included no sexual intercourse until the incision heals. Her husband's response to the nurse was, "My wife has not thought about sex in years." Melba is to have home visits from a registered nurse.

Case Study

The home health agency nurse arrives at Melba's home. After introducing herself, the nurse begins to take Melba's vital signs, but finds it hard to concentrate as Melba wants to talk about her prior health problems and surgeries. Melba describes a series of surgeries and complaints going back several years beginning at age 26 with back surgery, although she is somewhat lacking in details of what was found or done in the surgery. Then there was the time she could not seem to empty her bladder: "It would fill up with nearly a gallon before I could get somewhere to be catheterized." Melba describes excruciating pain when urinating, bladder infections, and high fevers off and on for several years. Her health care provider has not diagnosed any bladder problems. She also talks about years of impaired coordination and balance keeping her from being able to work. Melba says sometimes she can't sleep at night because it feels like ants are crawling under her skin. She currently complains of knee pain keeping her from walking. X-rays and an MRI of the knee were negative. From Melba's story, the nurse feels certain that there have been few or no periods of time in Melba's life that she has been symptom-free. The nurse finishes the vital signs, which are normal, and suggests Melba learn to do the wet to dry dressings for her abdominal incision. Melba says her husband will do the dressings and to teach him. The nurse recalls an old lecture from nursing school and realizes that some of Melba's behavior sounds like it matches what she learned about Somatization Disorder.

Questions

1. What is Somatization Disorder? What symptoms does Melba have or has she had that caused the nurse to think she might have Somatization Disorder? Could a person have some symptoms of this disorder and not meet the criteria for the diagnosis?

2. How do you think you might feel if you were working with Melba or a client with a similar history of physical complaints for which no medical explanation can be found?

3. What are the current theories about the causation of Somatization Disorder?

4. What is the incidence of Somatization Disorder?

5. Do nurses other than psychiatric nurses need to know about this disorder, and if so, where would nurses encounter a client with this diagnosis or some of the traits of this disorder?

6. If you were Melba's nurse, how would you respond when she tells you that she is not going to learn to do the dressing change and that you can teach her husband to do it?

7. What assessment areas would you like to assess if you were this client's nurse?

Questions (continued)

8. What impact might culture have on a client's symptoms?

9. What nursing diagnoses would you most likely write for this client? What would be some treatment goals of the nurse and client? What interventions would seem indicated for this client and possibly for the majority of clients with Somatization Disorder?

10. What are current treatment approaches to clients with this disorder?

Amanda

GENDER

Female

AGE

34

SETTING

- Adult psychiatric unit

ETHNICITY

- White American

CULTURAL CONSIDERATIONS

- Rural southern farming and strong churchgoing culture
- Culture of abuse

PRE-EXISTING CONDITION

CO-EXISTING CONDITION

COMMUNICATION

DISABILITY

SOCIOECONOMIC

- Raised poor then lower middle class when married

SPIRITUAL/RELIGIOUS

- Subconscious resistance to church related to abuse history.

PHARMACOLOGIC

PSYCHOSOCIAL

- Alternates between being withdrawn and uninhibited based on what alternative personality ("alter") is in charge.

LEGAL

- Need to avoid causing false memories of abuse
- Confidentiality

ETHICAL

- Is it educational or is it inappropriate, exploitive, and unethical to ask a client with Dissociative Identity Disorder (DID) to appear in public to discuss or demonstrate alternative personalities?

ALTERNATIVE THERAPY

PRIORITIZATION

DELEGATION

DISSOCIATIVE IDENTITY DISORDER (FORMERLY MULTIPLE PERSONALITY DISORDER)

Level of difficulty: High

Overview: Requires knowledge of DID and critical thinking to respond therapeutically to the client and any "alters," which present with a variety of behaviors and attitudes. Requires critical thinking to avoid letting personal attitudes or feelings get in the way of working effectively with the client and to avoid leading the client to false memories.

DIFFICULT

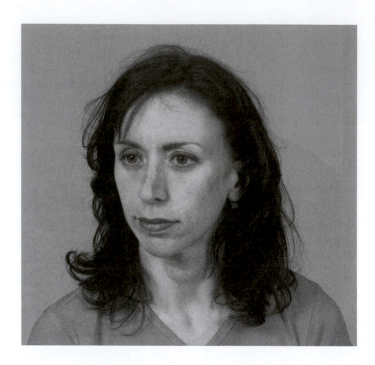

Client Profile

Amanda is a 34-year-old married female who was raised in a strong church-going family on a rural southern Bible Belt farm. Her grandfather as well as her father sexually, physically, and mentally abused her as a child. Each of them told her it would kill her mother if she found out and not to tell anyone or they would punish her. Her father, a deacon in the church, routinely abused her on Sundays after church and Sunday dinner when other family members took a nap. At first Amanda screamed, but no one seemed to hear. She began to dissociate: to mentally float above what was happening and feel like an observer. Her grandfather and her father died before she was 10 years old. Amanda repressed the abuse in her subconscious mind. At age 19 Amanda married Fred, a long-distance truck driver, who was kind to her but not often home. The marriage provided a means to get away from her mother who wasn't kind or supportive and who had actually known about the abuse and done nothing.

Recently Amanda noticed what she calls "trashy" clothes in her closet. She thought her husband had bought the seductive dresses until she found a charge receipt with her signature on it. Amanda has found herself in a store temporarily unable to recall what she came to buy or who she is. She has found herself talking in a strange childish voice or in a sultry seductive way: not like her real self at all. Amanda suspects she has different personalities within herself: one (Audrey) who likes to dress "trashy," tease men, and control; a small playful bear ("Bear"); "Sissy," age 5, who likes to play but is afraid of adults; Tom, who knows about "Sissy" and wants to protect her. Neither Tom nor Sissy know about Audrey, who seems to know everyone except Butch, who is angry about the abuse and wants Amanda to cut her arms. Amanda never has felt connected to the world and other people. She has little recall of her childhood and tries to deny flashbacks of the abuse.

Case Study

Amanda is admitted to the adult psychiatric unit. Her husband tells the nurse he fears his wife is " going crazy." Fred describes Amanda cutting her arms and having periods of time for which she has no memory. He relates that Amanda became very upset when he asked her to go to church with him. After the husband leaves, the psychiatric technician goes through the things Amanda brought to the hospital and removes items that she might hurt herself with, inventories them, and locks them up. The admitting orders provide a diagnosis of Dissociative Identity Disorder. The psychiatrist's history and physical on Amanda states she has had one previous admission to the facility. The nurse orders and reads the old chart from medical records and becomes aware of some of the alters (alternative personalities) Amanda has revealed to her psychiatrist and therapists. The nurse offers to play checkers with Amanda after the evening meal. During the checker game one of the alters comes out and says in a child's voice, "I don't want to play with you."

Questions

1. If you were the nurse on the unit, what would you say to the husband when he says that his wife (your client) is "going crazy"?

2. Why is the diagnosis of DID controversial? Is this a real disorder, or do mental health professionals and clients misapply and misuse this diagnosis?

3. What is the culture of abuse? What role did the southern, rural farm, Bible Belt culture possibly play in the abuse and dissociation?

4. Are all clients who are diagnosed with DID survivors of sexual abuse, and are all sexual abuse survivors likely to have or to develop DID?

5. Discuss some characteristics and behaviors of a person with Dissociative Identity Disorder. What are the criteria for a diagnosis of DID, and does Amanda meet the criteria for this diagnosis?

6. What is the cause of DID? What are the risk factors for DID?

7. If you were the nurse playing checkers with Amanda and she said in a childlike voice, "I don't want to play with you," what therapeutic response would you make and why?

8. What should the nurse do if the treatment team doesn't want staff nurses to interact with the client's alters?

9. Are alters real people within one person's body?

10. Why do people who have DID self-mutilate? If you were Amanda's nurse, how would you respond to this client or any client who is thinking of hurting herself, threatening to hurt herself, or has hurt herself?

11. What nursing diagnoses and treatment goals might the nurse write for this client?

12. What are some of the nursing interventions and professional treatment approaches to DID?

13. What additional research is being done in the area of DID?

GENDER	**SPIRITUAL/RELIGIOUS**
Female	
AGE	**PHARMACOLOGIC**
31	
SETTING	**PSYCHOSOCIAL**
Physician's office	
ETHNICITY	**LEGAL**
White American	■ Need to avoid libel or slander
CULTURAL CONSIDERATIONS	**ETHICAL**
	■ Refusing to treat client or alienating client so she goes to another health provider is questionable from an ethical standpoint
PREEXISTING CONDITION	
	ALTERNATIVE THERAPY
COEXISTING CONDITION	■ Getting a pet
	■ Volunteer work
COMMUNICATION	**PRIORITIZATION**
DISABILITY	**DELEGATION**
SOCIOECONOMIC	
■ Has a trust fund and is upper class without having to work	

FACTITIOUS DISORDER

Level of difficulty: High

Overview: Requires keeping an open mind while carefully observing and assessing client's behaviors and sharing findings with team members who must be consistent in their responses to the client. The nurse must control any negative thoughts or reactions and select an appropriate professional attitude and behaviors. Knowledge of transference and countertransference is useful. Avoidance of defamation of character by libel or slander is essential.

DIFFICULT

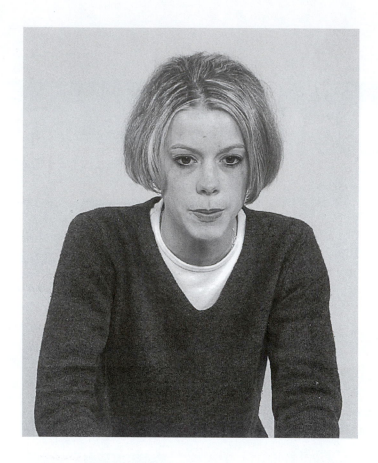

Client Profile

Linda is a 31-year-old single female who does not have to work as she has a trust fund left to her by a grandfather. A lawyer manages the trust fund and approves requests from Linda for money. Linda has lived in her own home, but is currently living with her parents because she says she is too ill at times to care for herself.

Linda has recently begun to frequently complain of seeing blood in her urine and having chills, fever, and bladder pain. She has been seeing a health care provider who is puzzled by her symptoms because the urinalyses are almost always normal with an occasional urine infection that responds to antibiotics. The client has a fever at each visit and looks pale and uncomfortable. On the first visit with the bladder-related symptoms, she provided a story about having extra pockets in her bladder wall that fill with urine and get infected; when they don't have urine in them, they have air, which is painful and requires hospitalization. In trying to verify this strange condition, the health care provider sought to find the name and address of the provider who identified it. The client was evasive, complaining of not remembering and providing a long involved story of earlier treatment by a urologist in a famous university hospital without supplying any real details.

Case Study

The office nurse goes to the waiting room to get Linda, weighs her, and takes her vital signs and a short history in preparation for seeing the health care provider. The nurse puts a glass thermometer in Linda's mouth and leaves the room to get a drink for the client who has complained of being thirsty. After the nurse closes the door, she remembers she forgot to remind the client to keep the thermometer under her tongue. As she opens the door, she thinks she sees the client take the thermometer from under the water faucet. The client quickly tells a story of needing to wash her hands. Linda's temperature is 101.8.

Although she cannot be sure the client had the thermometer under the faucet, the nurse mentions her suspicions to the health care provider. The provider does not say anything to the client but goes ahead with his assessment, and examination and orders a urinalysis. He tells the client he will be back after she is dressed. The doctor tells the nurse to recheck the temperature and stay in the room while it is being taken. The temperature is 98.4 on rechecking it. Neither the nurse nor the health care provider questions the client about this temperature. It is simply noted. The client is to drink at least six glasses of water a day and two glasses of cranberry juice and return in one week for further testing.

Later the health care provider mentions to the nurse in private that he suspects this client has Factitious Disorder. The provider tells the nurse he would like her to get some medical history on the client from the parents. The nurse recalls that she overheard the client tell the parents that the provider said he would have to run more tests and she was lucky to have parents to take care of her since she was so ill.

Questions

1. What is Factitious Disorder (FD), and how does this disorder differ from the somatoform disorders?

2. What do you suppose the nurse was thinking when she opened the door and thought she saw the thermometer being held under the faucet water by the client? What emotions might this observation arouse in the nurse?

3. Do you agree with the nurse's actions to say nothing of her suspicions about the thermometer being under the faucet to the client, but to then share her possible observation with the health care provider in private? Give a rationale for your answer.

4. If you were the nurse working with this client, how would you handle the situation if the provider asked you to recheck the client's temperature?

5. Does this client have any signs and/or symptoms that match the criteria for Factitious Disorder?

6. What is thought to be the cause of Factitious Disorder?

7. Why is the true incidence of Factitious Disorder in the general population unknown?

8. In what settings would a nurse encounter a client with Factitious Disorder?

9. If you were the nurse in this case, what additional assessments would you like to do? What nursing diagnoses would you likely find in this client or other clients with Factitious Disorder? What goals would you likely write for this client or other clients with Factitious Disorder?

10. What interventions would you likely write for this client or another client with a similar situation?

11. One of your peers asks you to explain Munchausen's Syndrome by Proxy. Give a brief explanation.

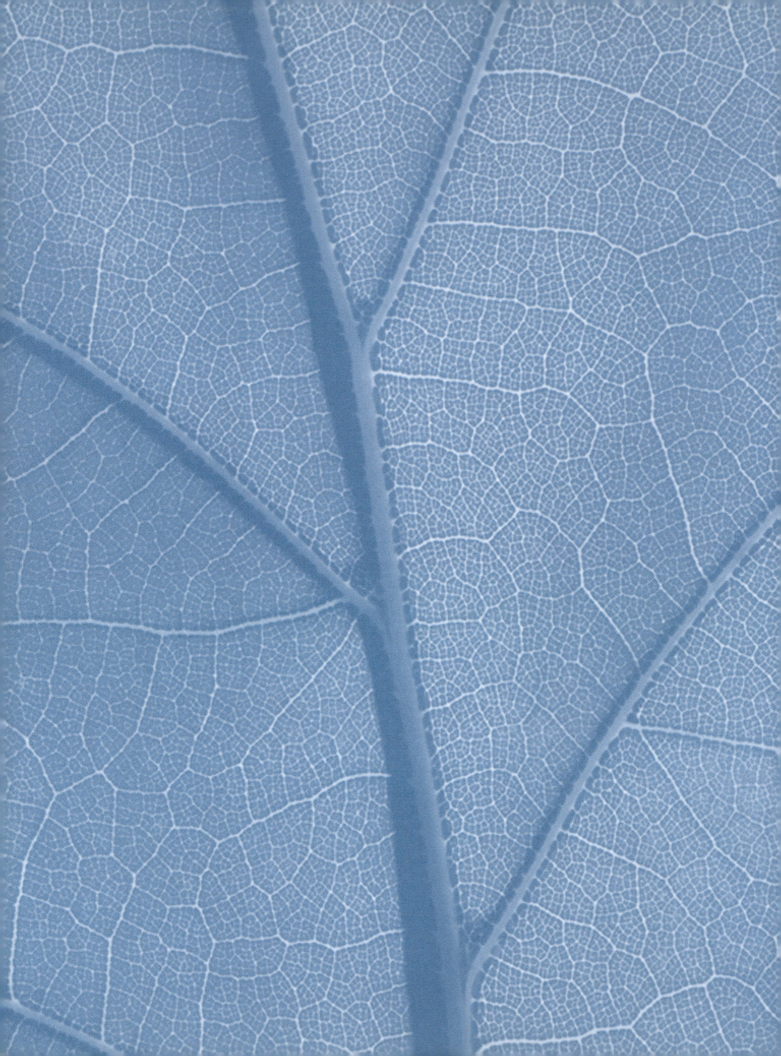

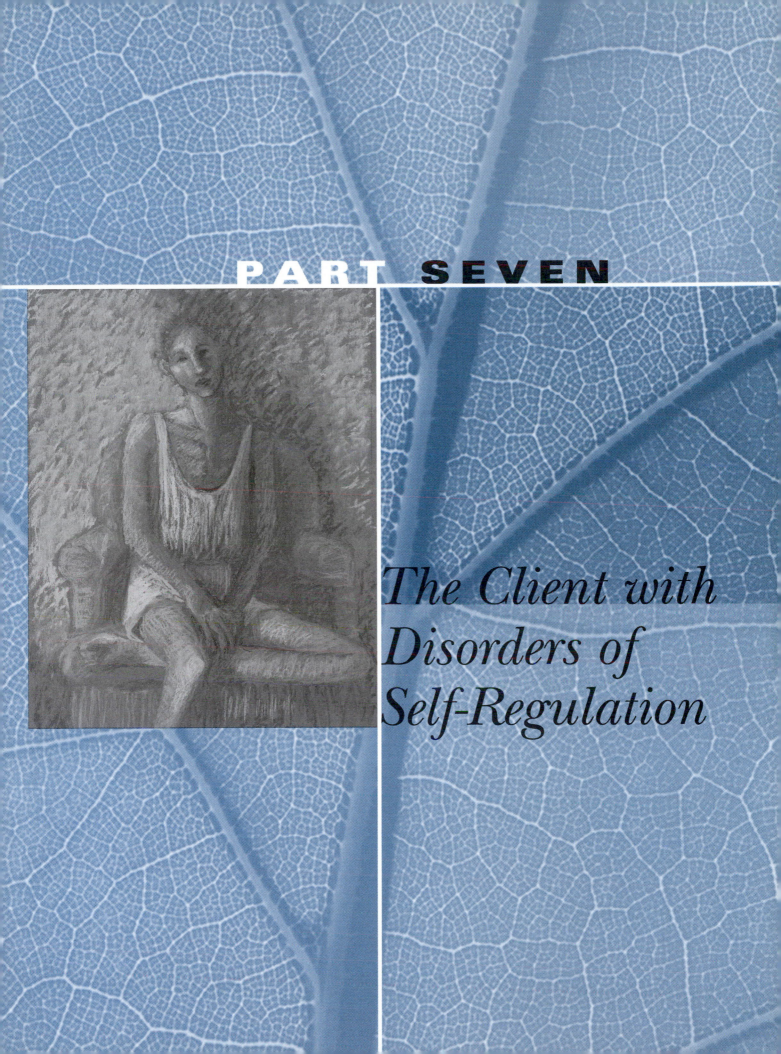

PART SEVEN

The Client with Disorders of Self-Regulation

GENDER

Female

AGE

26

SETTING

- Eating disorders unit of a private psychiatric hospital

ETHNICITY

- White American

CULTURAL CONSIDERATIONS

PREEXISTING CONDITION

COEXISTING CONDITIONS

- Nicotine abuse
- Alcohol abuse
- Depressed mood

COMMUNICATION

DISABILITY

SOCIOECONOMIC

- Upper middle class

SPIRITUAL/RELIGIOUS

- Connecting with a higher power to deal with abuse of food and alcohol and as a means of dealing with anxiety

PHARMACOLOGIC

- Buproprion hydrochloride (Wellbutrin, Zyban)

PSYCHOSOCIAL

- Socialization impaired by need to hide eating behavior

LEGAL

ETHICAL

ALTERNATIVE THERAPY

- Twelve-step program of AA for alcohol abuse and abuse of food
- Hypnosis for smoking

PRIORITIZATION

DELEGATION

BULIMIA NERVOSA, PURGING TYPE

Level of difficulty: Moderate

Overview: Requires knowledge of the signs and symptoms and behaviors associated with Bulimia Nervosa in order to identify clients who may have this disorder early on. Critical thinking is necessary to identify therapeutic approaches to clients with Bulimia Nervosa and to help them change harmful behaviors associated with binging and purging. Knowledge of the disorder is necessary in order to educate clients about the disorder.

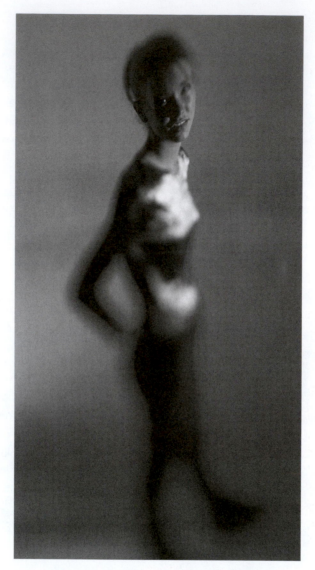

*Sabine has a distorted body image because of
her eating disorder.*

Client Profile   **Sabine** is a 26-year-old single woman who grew up in an urban upper-middle-class family in a western state. Her parents both worked and gave her whatever she wanted except their time, so she soothed herself with food. Sabine was a cheerleader in junior high school but failed to make the team in high school due to being overweight. Currently she is living alone in an apartment complex. She has a master's degree from a major university and earns over $100,000 a year managing a software development team. Sabine wants an attractive figure and will do almost anything not to be overweight like she was as a teenager. For the past four months, four or five times a week, she has been stopping at night at the grocery store on the way home from work and buying foods she has been denying herself in her previous dieting phase—donuts, cookies, potato chips, and ice cream bars—which she eats as fast as she can in the car on the way home. When she gets home she goes to the bathroom and makes herself vomit. She feels guilty after the binging and vows she won't do it again, but within a few days she finds herself binging again. She also eats excessively at all-you-can-eat buffets, then goes home and takes an excessive amount of laxatives and prune juice. Sabine feels guilty about her binging and purging, abuses alcohol to make herself forget, then feels guilty about drinking too much, and eats some more. She smokes from one to two packages of cigarettes a day. Sometimes she feels "depressed."

Sabine began to have abdominal discomfort and pain in the middle of her chest (esophageal area). She went to see a nurse practitioner, who noticed that she had enlarged parotid glands and eroded teeth enamel. When questioned about her eating habits, Sabine admitted to binging and purging. The nurse practitioner convinced Sabine to get treatment at an inpatient eating disorder program. Sabine went home, called work to arrange time off, drank a few drinks, packed a couple of suitcases, and called a taxi to take her to the eating disorders unit.

Case Study

Sabine is admitted to the eating disorders unit. During the initial assessment by the primary nurse, Sabine describes bowel irregularities and says she will need the laxatives she brought with her. The nurse advises Sabine that all the laxatives she has will have to be turned in and any she takes will have to be ordered by the doctor and dispensed by the nurse. Sabine becomes very upset and says: "I will talk to the doctor about this. I will just leave if I can't have my laxatives that I need."

The nurse reviews Sabine's chart and the CBC report, and during the initial assessment notices the client's affect is somewhat blunted. The nurse notices the client's enlarged parotid glands and the erosion of dental enamel. The nurse looks at Sabine's hands and asks: "Are you left-handed or right-handed?" Sabine answers: "Left-handed."

The nurse finds that Sabine weighs 142 pounds and is 5 foot 5 inches tall. Sabine sees herself in the mirror and says: "I look like a beer barrel." A psychiatrist, who examines Sabine, makes a diagnosis of Bulimia Nervosa. He orders individual and group therapy, a 12-step program, and buproprion hydrochloride (Wellbutrin). She asks for hypnosis to help with smoking cessation, and the psychiatrist orders it. After a few days, Sabine is offering to help on the unit.

Questions

1. What signs did the nurse practitioner and the nurse find that would lead any health care professional to suspect an eating disorder? What signs and symptoms suggest Sabine has Bulimia Nervosa and not Anorexia Nervosa? How do these eating disorders differ and how are they similar?

2. The psychiatrist gave Sabine a diagnosis of Bulimia Nervosa, Purging Type. What criteria does she have to meet to receive this diagnosis? Does she appear to meet these criteria?

3. Why was the nurse interested in knowing whether the client was left-handed or right-handed? When the nurse reviews the lab tests, which tests are likely to be abnormal in this client because of purging by self-induced vomiting?

4. What two screening questions could the nurse practitioner have used to screen this client for Bulimia? What other screening(s) might the nurse have done?

5. What possible reasons could the nurse practitioner have had for referring the client to an inpatient eating disorders clinic rather than an outpatient program?

6. What items might Sabine have brought with her to the hospital that would have to be inventoried and locked up? Can the nurse delegate these tasks to ancillary staff? How can the nurse deal with Sabine's threat to leave if she is not allowed to keep her laxatives?

Questions (continued)

7. Sabine offers to help the nurses with little tasks and in general tries to please the nurses on the unit. Is this common behavior of someone with Bulimia Nervosa, and what must you and other nurses keep in mind when this occurs?

8. You are teaching a class on the eating disorders unit. Sabine wants to know if males ever suffer from Bulimia Nervosa. She has observed that all the clients on the unit are female. Peers ask about the usual onset of Bulimia and the cause of Bulimia. How would you answer these questions?

9. Clients with Bulimia who are in the education class about the disorder, learn about medical problems that arise from their binging and purging. What medical problems associated with Bulimia Nervosa do these clients, nurses, and other health care professionals need to be aware of?

10. When assisting in gathering data on this client, what information would you especially be interested in gathering?

11. What nursing diagnoses would Sabine likely have that are related to her diagnosis of Bulimia Nervosa? What goals would you likely write for this client?

12. What interventions would you need to write and implement for this client? What interventions would you need to be sure and include with this client. What nonpharmaceutical interventions are commonly used with clients who have Bulimia Nervosa? Are medications used to treat Bulimia Nervosa? What are the likely reasons for the health care provider ordering buproprion hydrochloride (Wellbutrin, Zyban)?

Deidre

GENDER

Female

AGE

21

SETTING

- General hospital

ETHNICITY

- East Asian American mother and
  White American father (deceased)

CULTURAL CONSIDERATIONS

- Eastern value of honesty conflicts with
  need to hide and lie about hair pulling

PREEXISTING CONDITION

COEXISTING CONDITION

- Depressed mood

COMMUNICATION

DISABILITY

SOCIOECONOMIC

- Low-income college student with
  scholarship and part-time job with
  little or no help from family

SPIRITUAL/RELIGIOUS

PHARMACOLOGIC

- Fluoxetine (Prozac)

PSYCHOSOCIAL

- Prior sexual abuse
- Isolates herself to pull hair

LEGAL

- Adult client reveals sexual abuse
  as a child

ETHICAL

ALTERNATIVE THERAPY

- Marjoram Leaves
- Aromatherapy
- Acupuncture
- Hypnosis

PRIORITIZATION

DELEGATION

IMPULSE CONTROL DISORDERS: NOT ELSEWHERE CLASSIFIED TRICHOTILLOMANIA

Level of difficulty: Moderate

Overview: Requires knowledge of impulse control disorders, understanding of the client's background and personal situation, empathy and rapport with the client, and understanding of the impact of traditional and alternative medications and therapies.

Client Profile

Deidre is a 21-year-old student at a large university, on scholarship and part-time work with little financial help from her family. When she was seven, her mother went into the psychiatric hospital for depression. Her father had been killed in an accident when she was a toddler so a grandfather cared for Deidre and her brother. The grandfather sexually abused her, and by the time her mother came home Deidre literally was pulling her hair out. She would pull first one hair and then another from the top of her head and then eat the hair. Deidre also pulled out eyelashes at times and began to pull out pubic hair, thinking no one would see that area and she could better hide her hair pulling. She did not tell her mother about the sexual abuse because her grandfather said her mother would either go away again or die if she found out. Deidre isolates herself, choosing not to date or go places with other girls. She tries hard not to pull her hair out and may go several days without pulling, but always begins again. Her habit is to carefully choose a hair, twirl the hair, pull it in such a way as to remove the hair bulb with the hair, rub the hair between her fingers, and then eat it.

Case Study

Deidre has been eating marjoram leaves and doing aromatherapy in an effort to stop eating hair. She experiences a loss of appetite, weight loss, weakness, diarrhea, nausea and vomiting, increased white blood cells, and fever. She has resisted going to see a health care provider, but finally allows her mother to take her to the provider's office. The provider notices Deidre has a strange pattern of baldness on her head. He asks her if she pulls her hair, but she denies it. Deidre is admitted to the hospital for observation prior to possible exploratory laparoscopy. The primary nurse assigned to Deidre does a head-to-toe assessment and makes a note of the bald spot at the top of Deidre's head. Later the nurse forgets to knock before entering Deidre's room, and just as she is getting ready to apologize for not knocking, she sees Deidre, with her eyes closed, put what looks like a hair in her mouth and swallow it. During the hospitalization, Deidre undergoes an exploratory laparoscopy. The surgeon finds a trichobezoar. When the surgeon confronts Deidre about the trichobezoar, the mother becomes angry with Deidre for insisting on the first visit to the health care provider and thereafter that she was not eating her hair. Deidre's mother demands that Deidre stop eating hair and stop lying immediately.

The health care provider diagnoses Deidre with Trichotillomania, suggests acupuncture and hypnosis, and prescribes fluoxetine (Prozac).

Questions

1. Why do you suppose Deidre denied pulling her hair when the health care provider asked her? Is it common for people who pull their hair out to deny it?

2. What is Trichotillomania, and what are the essential features of Trichotillomania? Describe some common behaviors carried out by individuals with Trichotillomania.

3. You have entered the client's room without knocking. You are pretty sure that the client is not aware that you entered the room and saw her eating a hair. What will you do now? If you confront the client and she says: "You must be mistaken. I would never think of doing such a thing," what do you say or do?

4. Is there a relationship between Trichotillomania and self-esteem and/or body image?

5. What is a trichobezoar? Is the response of the mother, to the news that Deidre has a trichobezoar, helpful or not? How will you respond to the client and her mother in regard to what the mother has said to the client?

Questions (continued)

6. Deidre's mother asks you, "What causes Trichotillomania?" and "What are the complications of Trichotillomania?" What is your response?

7. What happens when people with Trichotillomania try to just stop pulling their hair as Deidre's mother suggests?

8. The client asks you if you think munching marjoram leaves and some aromatherapy will calm her enough to stop the impulses to pull out her hair. What will you tell her? What type of treatment has been found to work for people with Trichotillomania? Discuss acupuncture and hypnosis as treatments for Trichotillomania.

9. What teaching will you do on fluoxetine (Prozac)? What response will you give to the client sharing her fear she cannot afford the Prozac?

10. What is your response to the client's revelation that she was sexually abused when she was seven years old and she wants to keep it a secret?

11. What do you think is the primary nurse's role in caring for this client?

12. Based on the information you have, what nursing diagnoses, goals, and interventions would be appropriate for this client?

GENDER

Male

AGE

25

SETTING

Pediatric unit then local jail

ETHNICITY

- White American

CULTURAL CONSIDERATIONS

- Small town, large family

PREEXISTING CONDITION

COEXISTING CONDITION

COMMUNICATION

DISABILITY

SOCIOECONOMIC

- Lower middle class

SPIRITUAL/RELIGIOUS

PHARMACOLOGIC

PSYCHOSOCIAL

- Isolation due to stigma and fear of being found out
- Stress on marital relationship due to past and current sexual contact with children

LEGAL

- Reporting requirements in regard to a child telling about sexual activity with an adult
- Acting on sexual urges with children is a crime and punishable by law

ETHICAL

- Do Pedophiles deserve treatment and compassion or just punishment such as incarceration, probation, lifelong tracking, and ostracism?

ALTERNATIVE THERAPY

PRIORITIZATION

- Safety of the child
- Safety of other children (future victims)
- Need for psychological and medical help for child as victim as well as for child's family
- Psychological and other treatments for the client as perpetrator
- The perpetrator needs to be kept safe from hurting others and safe from suicide attempts

DELEGATION

PEDOPHILIA

Level of difficulty: High

Overview: Requires the ultimate in professionalism to help a person who has Pedophilia learn to control their sexual urges and to live in society without being sexually involved with children. Involves reporting to a state agency any information provided by children who have been the subject of sexual acts or personal knowledge of sexual activities between a child and an adult. Requires ability to assess for suicidal ideation and to "anchor" a person who has suicidal potential.

DIFFICULT

Client Profile

Edgar, a 25-year-old married male with a stepdaughter and a natural daughter, grew up the youngest child in a large family. The family lived in a small town where everyone knew everyone, but there were secrets in Edgar's family. Edgar's father drank a lot and talked about sex a lot, and something did not seem right when he was around small children. A couple of his grown children would not trust him alone with their children.

When Edgar graduated from high school, he moved into his married sister's home. In the car one day, her 6-year-old son said something that caused her to suspect sexual activities between her brother and her son. She had no proof, but she asked Edgar to leave. Edgar immediately moved in with his brother's family. He shared a room with the brother's 5-year-old boy. Edgar's brother had no idea of what had transpired in the sister's home. Not too long after Edgar moved in, his brother was playing with his son and the son asked if he wanted to play "tiger bellies" like Uncle. When he was asked what that was, the boy's father was shocked to hear it involved some genital stimulation. Edgar admitted to his brother that he had experienced fantasies and sexual urges about sex with children since he was 16 years old. Edgar was asked to leave and told by his brother to get counseling. Edgar did not go to counseling, but instead found himself another place to stay and a well-paying job. Within a couple of months, he married an attractive woman who had a 3-year-old daughter and a year later they had another child.

Case Study

Edgar's 5-year-old daughter, Mindy, is in the hospital for treatment associated with her diabetes. The hospital is in the closest city to the small town where the family lives. Edgar is going to stay all night on the cot in the child's room while his wife stays at home with the other daughter. The night nurse makes rounds and finds Mindy sleeping on the cot with Edgar. The night nurse did not think too much about this as children often feel insecure in the hospital and want their parents close by. The next day Mindy says to her primary nurse: "Don't touch me down there. Only my daddy can touch me there. Oops, I am not to tell anyone. Don't tell anyone, please."

Edgar finds himself in jail waiting to see the judge in regard to child sexual abuse charges. His wife has threatened divorce. He has begged her not to divorce him. He has agreed to go into treatment, yet he is afraid he will be sent to prison and lose his wife, his job, and all respect from any source due to the stigma attached to sexual preference of children and child molestation. The nurse working at the jail makes rounds. The nurse is to do a brief check on this new inmate.

Questions

1. What actions had to taken in response to Mindy's revelation that her daddy is the only one who can touch her "down there" (her genitals) in a certain way?

2. Does Edgar's behavior match the diagnostic criteria for Pedophilia? Does a person who meets these criteria have to experience distress in some area of functioning to have the diagnosis of Pedophilia? Do most Pedophiles abuse only children in their family or belonging to friends or neighbors?

3. Are some Pedophiles attracted only to children of a certain age? Do most Pedophiles begin to have sexual urges, fantasies, or activity with children in adolescence like Edgar? What justification do people with Pedophilia use when they have sexual activity with a child or children?

4. Is it unusual that this client is married, has sex with his wife, and has a second child? Are all Pedophiles male like the client in this case?

Questions (continued)

5. What are the current beliefs about the cause(s) of Pedophilia? Are all child abusers Pedophiles?

6. What did you think or feel when you read that Edgar had sexual activity with two of his nephews and then his stepdaughter?

7. Edgar was advised by his brother to go into counseling for his unacceptable behavior with children. Were you surprised that he didn't go to counseling? Why or why not?

8. If you were the nurse working in the jail, what would you ask Edgar and/or tell him when you go to do a brief check on him?

9. Will Edgar go to prison and/or to treatment, and will he have to register as a sexual offender?

10. Can Pedophilia be treated, and if so, what kinds of medications, therapy, and other treatments are being used today to treat Pedophiles?

11. Where will nurses encounter and care for people with Pedophilia in addition to pediatric units and the jail, and what will their role be?

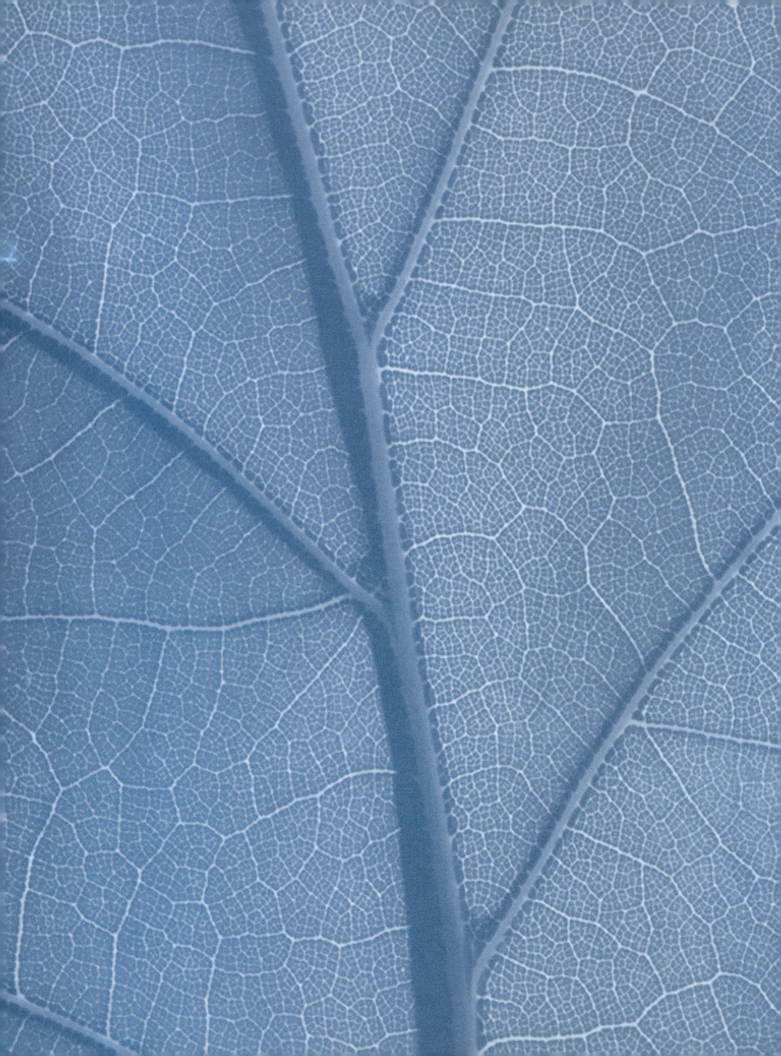

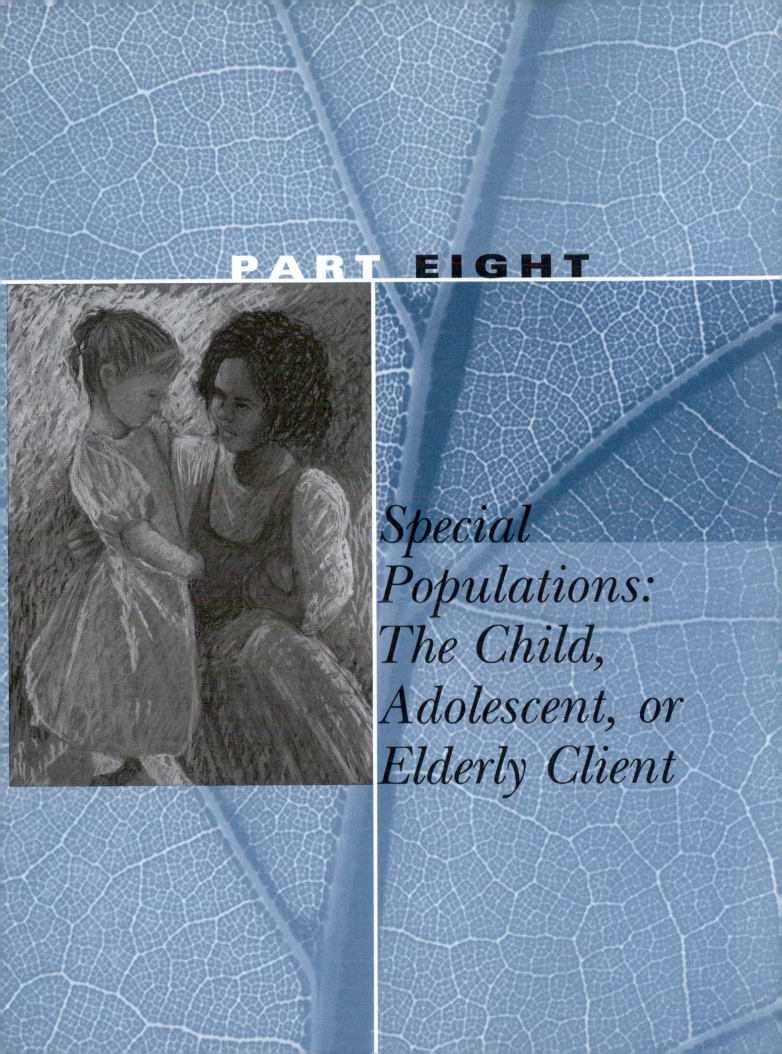

PART EIGHT

Special Populations: The Child, Adolescent, or Elderly Client

Len

GENDER

Male

AGE

13

SETTING

- Residential treatment facility for adolescents

ETHNICITY

- White American

CULTURAL CONSIDERATIONS

PREEXISTING CONDITIONS

COEXISTING CONDITIONS

COMMUNICATION

DISABILITY

SOCIOECONOMIC

- Parents divorced; mother is low income and father is middle income

SPIRITUAL/RELIGIOUS

PHARMACOLOGIC

PSYCHOSOCIAL

- Priority is being seen as tough by male acquaintances
- Difficulty establishing peer relationships

LEGAL

- History of sneaking out past legal curfew and drinking with older boys
- Found in neighbor's house uninvited; neighbor could press charges if Len leaves treatment early
- History of tardiness and skipping school

ETHICAL

ALTERNATIVE THERAPY

PRIORITIZATION

DELEGATION

MODERATE

OPPOSITIONAL DEFIANT DISORDER

Level of difficulty: Moderate

Overview: Requires working collaboratively as part of a multidisciplinary team, including client and client's family, to change the behavior of the client (a child) who has difficulty with authority figures. The nurse must be able to set limits consistently and help the client's family to recognize the need for, and to set, consistent limits for the child.

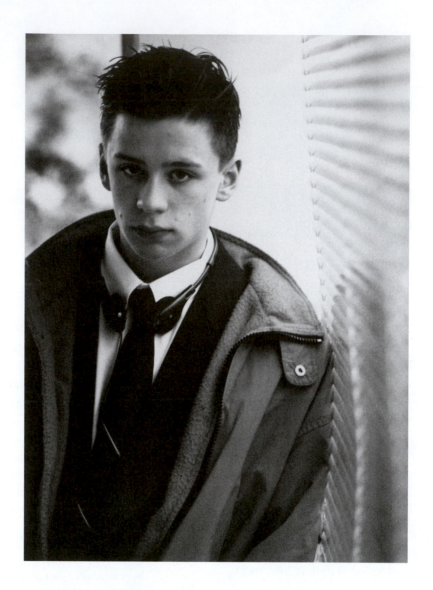

Client Profile

Len is a 13-year-old boy whose parents are divorced. Len's father is remarried and has two children by his second wife. The father is a truck driver and home only periodically. Len's mother tries to compete with his father in giving Len and his younger brother Nathan (Nate) material things. The mother recently bought Len some outrageously expensive tennis shoes that he demanded she buy. The mother doesn't work and has been buying things for Len and his brother on her brother's credit card. She is running up a large credit card debt on her brother's account and refuses to let him look at the bills that come in the mail. The boys and their uncle live with their mother, who is not good at setting limits. Their uncle and their father are also poor at setting limits.

Len has been in and out of trouble at school for the past year. He curses in class and is argumentative with teachers and the vice principal of his middle school. His mother takes Len's side in any disagreement between Len and authority figures. Len tells her that these adults are unfairly picking on him or they are stupid, and his mother believes him or at least she seems to when she goes to the school to "straighten the school people out." Recently a neighbor returned home to find Len in his house with some bizarre story of why he was there. The neighbor called the police who took Len into custody. The neighbor dropped charges when he learned that a deal had been worked out for the school system and Len's father's insurance to pay for Len going into residential psychiatric treatment.

Case Study

Len is admitted to a unit for adolescent boys at a residential treatment center by the nurse on duty. The nurse shows Len and his mother around the unit and gives both of them a copy of the unit rules. The nurse goes over the rules and has Len sign a statement that he has read, understands, and will abide by the rules. Consequences of breaking various rules are on the document. The unit is on a level system in which residents are promoted to a higher level and granted more privileges as they comply with rules and treatment. The nurse notices Len crossing his fingers, rolling his eyes, and then winking at his mother before signing the document.

Len and his mother are introduced to a nurse clinical specialist in child and adolescent mental health (certified by the American Nurses Association and prepared at the master's level in nursing) who will be Len's case manager, individual therapist, and the family therapist. Case managers in this facility can be nurse clinical specialists, master's prepared social workers or psychologists, or licensed professional counselors. The treatment plan is managed by the case manager but is developed, implemented, and evaluated by the treatment team members, from various disciplines, at formal meetings at designated time intervals.

Mother says to the nurse clinical specialist and the unit nurse: "I hope you will fix him so I can take him home soon. How soon can I visit?"

During the next few days, Len tests the staff by refusing to comply with unit rules, such as refusing to get out of bed and refusing to complete hygiene tasks without several prompts and using cuss words. Len loses his temper with peers and staff. Peers accuse him of hiding their belongings and playing pranks on them, which he denies and blames on someone else.

At a meeting of the staff in which Len's case is discussed, treatment team members from the various disciplines offer input about Len's behavior since admission. The psychiatrist suggests a diagnosis of Oppositional Defiant Disorder. Len and his mother meet with the treatment team. Len is given his diagnosis, and it is explained to him. His input and his mother's input are sought in regard to treatment goals and interventions. Len's response to the team is: "I am not oppositional and I am not defiant. You are all wrong and stupid."

Questions

1. If you were the nurse admitting Len to the unit, how would you respond to Len when he crosses his fingers, rolls his eyes, and winks at his mother before signing the rules agreement form? Give a rationale for your response.

2. How could you as a staff nurse develop some rapport with Len? How would you develop rapport and a trusting relationship with the client's family?

3. You are assigned to have a one on one with this client and he says he has nothing to say and you cannot make him talk. How would you react to this?

4. The health care provider asks you and the rest of the staff to identify behaviors in this client that match the diagnosis of Oppositional Defiant behavior. Does the client have behaviors that match the criteria for this disorder?

Questions (continued)

5. What if you as a staff nurse decide you don't like some of the interventions that the team has implemented and you would like to try something different? Can you do this?

6. One of the staff asks you: "What causes Oppositional Defiant Disorder?" What would you reply?

7. What nursing diagnoses would you write for this client? What goals would you write for this client?

8. Would you expect this child to be on medication to treat Oppositional Defiant Disorder? What interventions do you think would work with this client?

9. The client talks with his mother on the phone and convinces his mother that he is better and asks her to come get him. He has not been discharged. How would you convince the mother that her son is not ready to be discharged?

10. Is there a link between Oppositional Defiant Disorder and Conduct Disorder and is there a link between ODD and ADHD?

Brandon

GENDER

Male

AGE

14

SETTING

- Pediatric unit of hospital

ETHNICITY

- White American

CULTURAL CONSIDERATIONS

PREEXISTING CONDITION

COEXISTING CONDITIONS

- Seizure disorder and mild mental retardation

COMMUNICATION

DISABILITY

- Impaired social interaction

SOCIOECONOMIC

- Middle to upper-middle income family

SPIRITUAL/RELIGIOUS

PHARMACOLOGIC

- Carbamazepine (Tegretol)
- Vicodin

PSYCHOSOCIAL

- Withdraws from others
- Limited speech
- Poor social skills
- Dependent on parents for help with activities of daily living

LEGAL

- Need for informed consent to gather information from health care providers and others outside the hospital system

ETHICAL

ALTERNATIVE THERAPY

PRIORITIZATION

DELEGATION

AUTISTIC DISORDER

Level of difficulty: High

Overview: Requires using the usual caregiver as a resource in planning and implementing care for a child who has Autistic Disorder and does not relate well to people. Requires prioritization of clients and determination of tasks to be delegated.

Client Profile

Brandon is a 14-year-old boy who was diagnosed with Autistic Disorder just before his third birthday. His older sister Anne also has Autistic Disorder. Three other siblings do not have the disorder. As a toddler Brandon would go off by himself and when people tried to get near him, he would make flapping motions and strike out at them. He has always been sensitive to clothing touching him, refusing to wear any rough feeling or new clothing. When seasons change his mother has to hide Brandon's old clothes or he would insist on wearing winter clothing in summer and summer clothes in winter. Brandon loves to put pebbles or marbles in a container then take them out and put them back one by one. He plays with a piece of string, a rubber band, or a small stick for hours. Brandon did not have very many words or sounds until he was enrolled in an early childhood education program prior to going to preschool. The speech therapist and teachers' aides worked very hard with him until he had sufficient vocabulary to make some of his needs known and to communicate in simple words and to give a hug to people who are familiar to him. He can use a message board if someone holds his elbow in a certain way. He exhibits echolalia. Brandon does not make eye contact with others, and sometimes people say he looks like he is in his own world. The teachers and mother get his attention by holding his face up or pinching his arm and using behavior modification rewarding techniques for his doing or saying what they are asking of him. Brandon sometimes rocks his body in a stereotypical fashion. He gets very upset when things are moved around in his room, his home, or in the classroom. Brandon plays tee-ball in a special league for kids with special needs, and he is very proud of his tee-ball uniform. He collects baseball cards and has them in a certain order. If they are out of order, he works hard to get them back in order. He often uses headphones and listens to music.

Brandon is a big boy for his age, nearly 6 feet tall, 200-plus pounds, and muscular. He is difficult to handle when he is upset. His mother is a petite women, and she has gotten a few bruises when interacting with Brandon and has had to stop the car sometimes when Brandon was pulling her hair or throwing things in the car. Brandon's father helps with Brandon when he is home, but the father travels with his job and is often away from home for several days.

Case Study

Brandon was practicing playing ball at home in the yard. His sister threw the ball in the street, and Brandon ran after it with his mother close behind yelling at him to stop. Brandon was hit by a car and taken by ambulance to the emergency room where he had a seizure and was moved to ICU for observation and treatment with Valium and an anticonvulsant. After about twenty-four hours he was moved to the pediatric unit of the hospital and admitted for further observation. He has a fractured radius, and his arm is scheduled to be casted in the morning. The pediatric nurse assigned to care for Brandon and admit him to the pediatric unit observes that he is clearly upset as he makes all kinds of sounds and is flapping his arms. Brandon won't let anyone come near him. This is problematic as the health care provider wants Brandon's forearm in a splint wrapped with an ace bandage, the lower arm elevated in a sling, and an ice pack applied. The provider also orders carbamazepine (Tegretol) two times a day, Vicodin for pain as necessary, and bed rest.

Brandon's mother is near hysterical and crying. She tells the pediatric nurse that the ambulance personnel did not want her to ride in the ambulance with Brandon, although she advised the ambulance personnel that they would soon wish she were with Brandon. She relates that the same thing happened in ICU at the hospital. The

ICU nurse did not want to have Brandon's mother stay with him in ICU without documentation she was the legal guardian. Within minutes of asking the mother to leave ICU, the ICU nurse assigned to Brandon came to get the mother to help her with Brandon. The mother did have to telephone Brandon's father and ask him to fax proof she is a legal guardian.

The pediatric nurse assigned to Brandon has been listening to Brandon's mother tell her story, but realizes that there are three other assigned clients as well as Brandon. The nurse is to give two pediatric clients their 9 A.M. medicines that are ordered and do a specific gravity on the urine of the third client. It is now 8:55 A.M. A preoperative medication must be given to a burn client at 9 A.M. prior to going to a whirlpool treatment. Brandon still needs his forearm wrapped and elevated in a sling with an ice pack. He gets upset and strikes out at the nurse (but misses) when the nurse tries to give him a hospital gown and asks him to put it on.

Questions

1. What is going on with the mother that she is near hysterical and crying, and what would be a good response if you were the nurse in this case?

2. Assuming you were the nurse in this case and looking at the clients assigned to you and their needs, what would be your first and second priorities? What sort of things would make Brandon's care a first priority to you? Could you delegate some of the tasks that you have to do, and if so, what and under what circumstances?

3. What is Autistic Disorder (AD), and does Brandon have behaviors that meet the criteria for AD? Do all children with AD have the same symptoms as Brandon?

4. How would you approach getting Brandon to wear the hospital gown and stay in bed? How would you get Brandon's splint on his arm and get it wrapped and put ice on it?

5. How would you figure out when Brandon is in pain and in need of a pain pill?

6. Brandon needs to urinate, and his mother wants to take him to the bathroom. She insists he will be upset if he urinates in the bed, and he won't understand the urinal. Brandon is on bed rest. How would you handle this situation?

7. Brandon's parents ask you several questions including: "What are the current theories about the cause of Autism?" "What is the prevalence/incidence of Autism, and is it more prevalent in one gender compared to the other or not?" "What is the usual onset of Autistic Disorder?" and "What disorders or medical problems are commonly associated with Autism?" What would you include in your answer?

8. Discuss any assessments you need to do. What nursing diagnoses and goals would you write for Brandon, and what interventions would you include in the plan of care?

9. What would you need to know, and want to make sure the mother knows, about carbamazepine (Tegretol)?

10. What research is being done in the field of Pervasive Developmental Disorders including Autism and Asperger's Disorder/Syndrome? Is there research into families in which than one child has an Autism Spectrum Disorder?

GENDER	
Female	

AGE

8

SETTING

- School nurse's office

ETHNICITY

- White American

CULTURAL CONSIDERATIONS

- American culture values independence

PREEXISTING CONDITION

COEXISTING CONDITION

COMMUNICATION

DISABILITY

SOCIOECONOMIC

SPIRITUAL/RELIGIOUS

PHARMACOLOGIC

PSYCHOSOCIAL

- No close relationships with peers due to fear something will happen to mother if not near mother

LEGAL

- School attendance

ETHICAL

- Forcing child to work through anxiety and go to school versus homeschooling and not distressing child

ALTERNATIVE THERAPY

PRIORITIZATION

DELEGATION

SEPARATION ANXIETY DISORDER

Level of difficulty: Moderate

Overview: Requires awareness of behaviors associated with Separation Anxiety Disorder in order to identify children at risk for this disorder The nurse must work cooperatively with the parent, teacher and others, as well as the child, to plan and utilize interventions to resolve issues associated with separation anxiety.

Client Profile

Christine is an 8-year-old female who becomes very anxious when separated from her mother. She refuses to go to school or to stay there. Christine clings to her mother and cries and begs her not to leave her in the morning when she takes Christine to school. Christine has not made friends with peers. Christine recently tried to stay overnight at the house of a girl who wants to be her friend. Within an hour of arriving at the girl's home, she began describing fears that something bad was going to happen to her mother, so she was permitted to call home several times. Each time she learned that everything was fine. She did not eat much at dinner, complaining she was allergic to everything or did not like it. At bedtime, she began to cry because she had forgotten her pillow from home and she wanted her mother to bring it or to go home and get it. About 2 A.M., when she called home again, her mother came to get her. Christine's mother describes her as like a shadow, saying that Christine won't let her out of her sight at home. Most nights she comes and gets into the parents' bed because she is fearful of not being close to mother. She hears a siren in the dark and thinks the ambulance is coming for her mother.

Case Study

Christine comes to the school nurse's office complaining of a stomachache and wanting her mother to come and get her and take her home. When the nurse calls the home, no one answers the phone. The school nurse offers to call the father at work and have him come and take her home. Christine says, "No, I don't want my father to come for me." Christine seems very upset until she recalls her mother was going to the dentist. The school nurse is aware that Christine has been falling behind her class in schoolwork due to having her mother come and get her and take her home from school two or three times a week. Christine asks the school nurse: "Would you please call the dentist's office to see if my mother is there and if she is all right? Could you ask her to come get me and take me home when she is finished at the dentist's office?" The nurse makes the call and then asks Christine if there has been a time in which her mother was sick or a time in which she worried about mom.

When the mother arrives at the school, she tells Christine that she can't keep taking her out of school and that she must learn to stay in school. When the nurse says: "It sounds like you are concerned that Christine stay in school," the mother replies: "Why wouldn't I be with the school truancy officer calling and coming to the house? Besides that she won't pass this grade if her attendance does not get better."

The mother asks the school nurse if she thinks Christine could have school phobia and wants to know if she should homeschool Christine.

When the nurse asks Christine's mother whether there was a time when she was sick and Christine worried about her, the mother shares that two years ago when Christine's sister was born, she was in labor for an extended time and then had to have a caesarian section. The sister was premature and had to remain in the hospital for a month. The mother had a number of complications, almost died, and also was in the hospital for three weeks. The nurse asks how long Christine has been like a shadow to her and worried about her. The mother answers that it has been about two years, although it has been worse since summer vacation ended six weeks ago.

Questions

1. What could you do instead of calling the mother to come get Christine? What would you do if you could not reach the mother?

2. Christine's mother has asked if Christine could have school phobia. How would you answer, and what is your rationale?

3. Could Christine have Separation Anxiety Disorder? Does her behavior match any of the criteria for Separation Anxiety Disorder?

4. Why does the nurse ask Christine and then her mother if there was a time when the mother was sick and Christine was worried about her mother?

5. What causes Separation Anxiety Disorder? What is the usual course of Separation Anxiety Disorder?

6. Christine's mother asks: "Are there many other children who have difficulty separating from their mothers at school age?" How would you answer her?

7. At what developmental stage (according to Erickson) is Christine, what are the tasks of this stage, and is she mastering these tasks? Christine's mother asks the school nurse if she should home-school Christine. What would you say to her if you were the school nurse?

8. What treatments have been found to be successful in reducing separation anxiety from major attachment figures?

9. From the information you have about Christine, what nursing diagnoses would you write for her? What are some reasonable goals for Christine?

10. What interventions do you think would work for this client, and how could you go about getting the mother and teacher(s) invested in initiating these interventions? How would you evaluate success of interventions?

Phyu

MODERATE

GENDER

Female

AGE

7

SETTING

- School nurse's office

ETHNICITY

- Asian American (Myanmar, formerly called Burma)

CULTURAL CONSIDERATIONS

- Military culture and Asian (Myanmar)

PREEXISTING CONDITION

COEXISTING CONDITION

- Possible Social Phobia

COMMUNICATION

DISABILITY

SOCIOECONOMIC

- Middle class

SPIRITUAL/RELIGIOUS

PHARMACOLOGIC

PSYCHOSOCIAL

- Shy and selective mute

LEGAL

ETHICAL

ALTERNATIVE THERAPY

PRIORITIZATION

DELEGATION

SELECTIVE MUTISM

Level of difficulty: Moderate

Overview: Requires enlisting the cooperation of the client's family, teacher, and peers to work together to help the client feel safe and motivated to talk out loud in a variety of settings and to a variety of people.

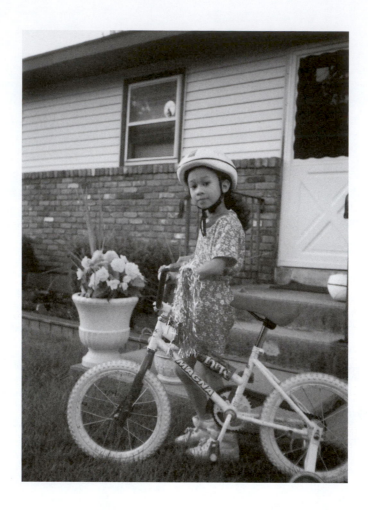

Client Profile

Phyu (pronounced Pee You) is 7 years old and lives with her mother and stepfather and an older sister. Her biological father lives in Myanmar (formerly Burma). Phyu's stepfather is a career military officer and currently on duty away from the family. The mother is from Myanmar. Phyu's mother and stepfather met in Bangkok where her mother had a job and the stepfather was on leave from the service. Phyu has moved frequently with her family, living first in Myanmar until her mother remarried, then on two different military bases in Asian countries. Recently the family moved to a small town in the Northwest near Phyu's stepfather's relatives while her stepfather was away on active duty.

Phyu has always been shy around distant relatives, strangers, and in strange situations. At 5 years old, she was talking to her sister in both English and the Myanmar language, but would not talk to anyone else. The parents and teacher did not worry about it the first month of school because they thought she was just shy and would start talking as soon as she got used to being in a different country and being at school. After the second month of not talking at school, the parents took Phyu to a pediatrician who diagnosed Phyu as having Selective Mutism. The parents thought Phyu would grow out of this problem, but it has persisted and now she is in the second grade and still does not talk in school.

Case Study

An older sister has brought Phyu to the school nurse's office. Phyu looks serious and somewhat sad. When the nurse asks her a question, Phyu plays with her hair, looks at the floor, and says nothing. The older sister talks for Phyu, saying that Phyu came to school this morning even though she was not feeling well and that she is now feeling worse and wants to go home. The school nurse starts to talk to Phyu, and her sister says: "She doesn't talk." The school nurse takes Phyu's temperature, and it is normal. Talking through the sister to Phyu, the school nurse learns that Phyu does not hurt anywhere but is "feeling bad." The school nurse asks Phyu and her sister to remain in the office and goes to talk briefly with the teacher. The teacher explains that the children in Phyu's class were going to be doing oral presentations, and a peer had teased her about her inability to talk in class and said: "I bet you won't give your report because the cat has got your tongue." Phyu was diagnosed with Selective Mutism when she was 5 years old, the teacher explains to the school nurse. The teacher says: "I would really appreciate it if you would work with me to find ways to help Phyu succeed at school. Perhaps you could get her mother involved in working with us. So far I have not had any luck getting the mother to participate in anything at school or to talk with me about Phyu on the phone."

Questions

1. If you were the school nurse, how would you respond to Phyu's request to go home?

2. You are the nurse in this case, and you decide to call the mother to come in and talk with you and the teacher. What action will you take if Phyu's mother offers a number of excuses for not coming to school to meet with you? What could be going on with the mother if she refuses to come to school for a discussion?

3. What is Selective Mutism? Which of the diagnostic criteria of Selective Mutism does Phyu meet?

4. When one of Phyu's teachers asks: "What causes Selective Mutism?" and "How common is Selective Mutism?" what will you tell him or her?

5. Does this client fit the usual pattern for age of onset of Selective Mutism? Is Selective Mutism found equally in boys and girls or not? What other disorders are frequently diagnosed concurrently with Selective Mutism?

6. What are children with Selective Mutism like?

7. What role do you think culture might play in this case?

8. What additional data would you like to gather on this child? What tentative nursing diagnoses would you likely write for this client? Working with Phyu's teachers and hopefully Phyu and her mother, what goals would be reasonable for Phyu?

9. What approach/interventions would you suggest to Phyu's mother, family, and teachers?

10. Why do you suppose some parents whose children have Selective Mutism don't want to get professional help for their children? Why do experts urge early diagnosis and treatment for children with Selective Mutism rather than waiting it out to see if it disappears?

11. In a conversation with the mother, she asks: "Is medication ever used to treat Selective Mutism, and if so, what medications?" How would you respond? What are the treatment approaches in addition to or instead of medication that are currently being used with children and adolescents?

Theera

GENDER

   Male

AGE

   5

SETTING

- Children's medical unit

ETHNICITY

- Asian American: parents born in Thailand and grandparents born in India

CULTURAL CONSIDERATIONS

- Culture of Thailand, including Buddhist religion and culture

PREEXISTING CONDITION

COEXISTING CONDITION

- Chronic constipation

COMMUNICATION

DISABILITY

SOCIOECONOMIC

- Parents recently finished graduate school; father has full-time work and mother has a part-time job

SPIRITUAL/RELIGIOUS

- Buddhist

PHARMACOLOGIC

PSYCHOSOCIAL

- Move from apartment to a house when child was age 2
- Followed by brief separation from parents

LEGAL

- Confidentiality issue

ETHICAL

ALTERNATIVE THERAPY

- Reflexology

PRIORITIZATION

DELEGATION

ENCOPRESIS

Level of difficulty: Moderate

Overview: Requires critical thinking/problem solving to develop rapport with a 5-year-old client and get him to voluntarily give up defecating in his underwear and to use the toilet for this purpose. Requires supporting not only the client but his parents, who are frustrated, angry, and embarrassed at times.

Client Profile

Theera is a 5-year-old boy who was born in the United States to parents from Thailand. His parents came to this country to attend graduate school, and that is where they met, married, and had Theera. When Theera was about 2 years old, they purchased a new home and moved from the apartment where they had lived all of Theera's life to a quiet suburban home. Soon after this family move, Theera's parents left on a business trip associated with the father's work and Theera was left in the care of extended family. Later, the mother's sister and her son, who is two years older than Theera, moved in with the family so she could attend college and help take care of Theera. At this time Theera was refusing to defecate in the commode in the bathroom, saying he would not do this until he went to school. He has had periods of passing small amounts of hard stool, usually about three times a week. Theera's mother has eagerly awaited the start of school, expecting he would defecate in the toilet; however, this has not happened. Once Theera began school, he started soiling his underwear and hiding it in various places in the school. The teacher began to discover the hidden underwear a little over three months ago and finally figured out it belonged to Theera when the mother, tiring of buying underwear because he never seemed to have any clean, decided to put labels in the underwear.

Case Study

Theera is admitted to the children's medical unit for a medical evaluation, which has revealed that although he has problems with constipation, the problem is not due to a medical condition. The primary nurse assigned to care for him reads Theera's psychosocial evaluation and learns the information in the profile above. In talking with the mother the nurse learns that the parents have been embarrassed that Theera still is not toilet trained. His room at home has been so odorous at times from hidden soiled underwear that they were embarrassed to have guests, and the cousin made fun of Theera being a baby. The father has been angry with the mother at times for not being able to make Theera use the toilet and "babying" him too much.

The mother shares that she has tried bribing Theera with promises of toys and that his father has tried spanking him to get him to use the toilet, all without success.

During a team meeting to do treatment planning for Theera, the nurse practitioner on the team says that she is building a somewhat conspiratorial relationship with Theera in which she has offered to help Theera hide his underwear. She has told Theera that he is not hiding them well enough and perhaps he could use her help to hide them better.

The nurse practitioner also shares reading about a social worker who has had good luck working with children with Encopresis to get them to not let the "poop" be the boss, much in the way children learn not to let bullies get the best of them. Some of the team members tell the primary nurse that they think these ideas are crazy and what this child needs is laxatives, suppositories, and/or enemas followed with bowel training as well as limit setting.

Questions

1. What are some common feelings nurses might have when working with a child who soils his underwear and hides it in inappropriate places like under his bed or in the dresser drawers? What are some responses that parents might have to a child with Encopresis?

2. What rationale could the nurse practitioner have had for offering to help Theera hide his underwear?

3. What are the criteria for a diagnosis of Encopresis, and do you think Theera meets these criteria?

4. You are teaching an in-service education on Encopresis for your peers. How would you respond to questions regarding the cause and incidence of Encopresis and how Encopresis relates to constipation and soiling?

5. What kinds of varied treatments are being utilized to treat children with constipation, and what treatments are used for Encopresis?

6. Define and discuss reflexology as a treatment for Encopresis.

7. Theera's Aunt comes to visit him. She asks you to tell her what the doctor has said about Theera's problem. She also tells you that she wants to give you some information about Theera and the family. What is your response to her request for information and her offer to give you information?

8. What do you think about the social worker's idea of talking to the child about being boss over the poop?

9. The mother mentions that she has gone to the Buddhist temple to take food and robes for the monks, light incense, and get a wish about Theera offered up to Buddha. She says she thinks this problem with his not going to the toilet may have something to do with Theera's past lives. What would be an acceptable response given that you are not of the Buddhist religion?

10. What nursing diagnoses and treatment goals would you likely write for Theera? What interventions do you think would be helpful for this child and his family?

Penny

GENDER	**SPIRITUAL/RELIGIOUS**
Female	
AGE	**PHARMACOLOGIC**
7	■ Desmopressin (DDAVP) tablets or spray
SETTING	**PSYCHOSOCIAL**
■ School nurse's office	■ Does not accept invitations for overnight stays from peers due to bedwetting
ETHNICITY	**LEGAL**
■ White American	
CULTURAL CONSIDERATIONS	**ETHICAL**
PREEXISTING CONDITION	**ALTERNATIVE THERAPY**
	■ Alarm to alert of wetness at night and behavior modification
COEXISTING CONDITION	■ Relaxation therapy
COMMUNICATION	**PRIORITIZATION**
DISABILITY	**DELEGATION**
SOCIOECONOMIC	

ENURESIS

Level of difficulty: Moderate

Overview: Requires an understanding of Enuresis and its possible causes. Requires patience, empathy, and ability to use creative thinking to develop interventions utilizing a knowledge of the way children think and behave according to their developmental level.

Client Profile

Penny is a 7-year-old girl who wets the bed at night, nearly every night, and has done so since she was a baby. Her father is upset with her because he says he is tired of the smell of urine-soaked sheets and her mother having to get up at night to help her change her bed. The father often drinks several beers after work at night. He tends to be angry with her when he is drinking. When he is drinking too much, he makes Penny get out of bed at night and wash her own wet bedsheets. Penny's father calls her lazy and stupid and says she will never learn to get out of bed and go to the bathroom at night and she won't ever have a boyfriend or a husband because no one wants a bed wetter.

Penny is upset with herself not only because of what her father says to her but also because she cannot stay overnight with anyone from school or have anyone stay overnight with her until she stops wetting the bed. Her self-esteem and confidence in herself is so low that she never tries to make friends. Penny stays dry during the day, but at night she awakes with her pajamas and bedsheets wet. Penny's mother wet the bed when she was Penny's age, but she has not talked with Penny about it as she is embarrassed and is afraid of her husband being angry. She feels guilty and ashamed about this secret.

Case Study

In school one day, Penny asks the teacher if she can go to the bathroom and the teacher asks her to wait until she finishes a spelling test. Penny wets her underpants and is sent to the school nurse's office to get cleaned up. The school nurse encourages Penny to talk about how she feels about wetting her underpants and then asks her if she realizes that this happens to lots of other children. The school nurse reveals that when she was a child, she wet her own bed at night for several years. Penny replies that this is the first time that she has wet her underpants in the daytime but that she does wet her bed at night too. She wishes that she could stop doing this, but she says she will probably wet her bed all her life because her father said she would. The school nurse offers to talk to Penny's parents and to try to get them to help her stop wetting the bed at night: "Please let me talk to them about helping you stop bedwetting. I believe you can stop the bedwetting. It may take some time and some work, but it can be done."

Questions

1. What is Enuresis? Are there subtypes of Enuresis?

2. If you were the school nurse and you had wet the bed as a child, would you share with a child that you had also wet the bed?

3. If you were the school nurse, how would you approach getting the parents to discuss what to do for Penny?

4. If Penny's parents refuse to meet with you and refuse to get her treatment, will her bedwetting at night resolve itself? What can Penny's parents and others like them try in order to resolve their child's bedwetting? Will this take a commitment on the part of the parents and mean a change in their behavior?

5. What is the usual course of Enuresis?

6. Does Enuresis typically run in families, and does it occur equally in both genders or in one more than the other? What is the incidence of Enuresis?

7. The parents do meet with you, and the father asks you "What causes bedwetting? Is it laziness?" What would you tell the father?

Questions (continued)

8. The mother asks if it is possible that Penny's bedwetting is due to a medical cause. How would you respond if you were the school nurse?

9. The parents would like to know if there is some treatment for bedwetting. The mother has heard that one of the neighbor children took some pills to stop it. What are the current treatments for Enuresis?

10. What assessment information would you like to have in order to write a nursing care plan on this client?

11. What nursing diagnoses and goals would you likely write for this client and her family? What nursing interventions would you likely initiate?

CASE STUDY 7

Hannah

GENDER

F

AGE

89

SETTING

- Home of client's daughter

ETHNICITY

- Black American

CULTURAL CONSIDERATIONS

PREEXISTING CONDITION

- Pernicious anemia

COEXISTING CONDITION

COMMUNICATION

- Requires hearing aides to hear

DISABILITY

- Difficulty hearing

SOCIOECONOMIC

- Upper middle class

SPIRITUAL/RELIGIOUS

- Methodist

PHARMACOLOGIC

- Anticholinergic medication
- Donepezil (Aricept)

PSYCHOSOCIAL

- Sits with old friends in Sunday school and with daughter in church: cannot recall events of the past or read bible verses but sings old familiar songs of her childhood

LEGAL

- Claiming power of attorney for a parent or declaring parent incompetent and getting guardianship

ETHICAL

- Ethical issue around making decisions for grown parents

ALTERNATIVE THERAPY

- Music therapy

PRIORITIZATION

DELEGATION

DEMENTIA OF THE ALZHEIMER'S TYPE

Level of difficulty: Moderate

Overview: Requires the nurse to be knowledgeable about Alzheimer's Disease and its stages. Nurse must do more explanations and teaching with the client's caregiver since the client has difficulty understanding or recalling what the nurse has explained to her. The nurse needs to determine when and if it is appropriate to see that the caregiver gets information about declaring the client incompetent or getting the power of attorney and about respite care.

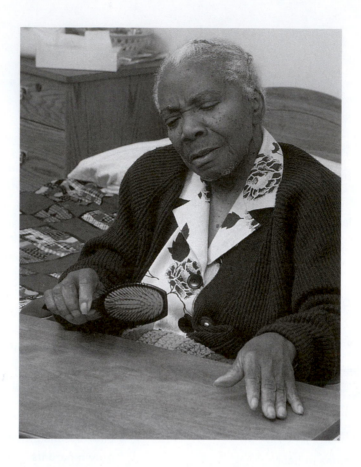

Client Profile

Hannah is an 89-year-old woman who had been living in her own home for years and fiercely protecting her independence from her five grown children. Hannah drove her car until she was 87 and did her own cooking, but had a cleaning woman come once a week. Women friends came on Sunday to take her to Sunday school and church. Hannah had been married three times, and one day in Sunday school she was asked to tell about her last husband who was now dead. She could not recall anything about him, including his name, so she said to a friend: "You tell about him." She did enjoy singing old familiar hymns and being with her women friends of many years. Hannah began to get even more forgetful, frequently forgetting the names of the grandchildren and her own children and covering this by calling them all "sugar." She began to pay some of her bills more than once, and when the daughter, Jean, found this out, she hired someone to live in with her mother and took over the bill paying. Jean decided to let her mother keep her car keys, but secretly took the battery out of the car. Hannah tried to start the car every day and would call Jean to tell her the car wasn't working, and Jean would say she had called someone to come repair it. The next day Hannah would forget that the car wasn't working and would try to start it again.

Within a week of Jean hiring someone to live with her, Hannah fired the woman. Jean decided to take her mother to live with her, about a ninety-minute drive from Hannah's home. Jean works out of her home and believed she could work and look after her mother without any problem; however, problems started as soon as Hannah arrived at Jean's home. Hannah begged people who called or came to visit her daughter to take her home. She would offer them money and say she was kidnapped. She fell and decided to stay in her bed and refused to get up. The daughter was unsure if her mother had broken her hip or not. Jean was concerned that her mother might be anemic because she had been diagnosed with pernicious anemia and was receiving B12 injections monthly before coming to live with Jean. Hannah lost five pounds after moving in with her daughter Jean. The weight loss was puzzling since her mother had a voracious appetite and seemed to eat enough for two people, demanding food several times a day in between meals and telling people "that woman is starving me." Jean decided to call a home health service that would send a home health nurse and a health care providers to the home and would draw blood for lab tests and send a mobile x-ray unit.

Case Study

A home heath agency nurse has come to visit Hannah at her daughter's home. Hannah offers the nurse a hundred dollars to take her home. Hannah whispers to the nurse that if she had car keys, she would drive herself home. The nurse fluffs up Hannah's pillows and chats with her awhile about her little dog. The nurse talks Hannah into letting him look at her hearing aids and check the batteries and into agreeing to wear the hearing aides. Hannah tells her daughter that she will wear the hearing aides "because that nice nurse wants me to wear them." After awhile the nurse gets Hannah to agree to have blood drawn for CBC, HIV, and thyroid tests. A portable X-ray technician is called to come and get an X-ray of Hannah's hip.

The nurse asks Jean if she has any old pictures of Hannah's parents or siblings and discovers a wedding picture of the parents. Hannah immediately identifies her parents. The nurse tests Hannah's orientation and finds she does not know the year, month, or day. Hannah thinks it is 1941. She refers to her daughter as "that woman who kidnapped me." The nurse does a Mini Multi-State Examination (MMSE).

The nurses talks to the client before leaving and tells her that a "nice doctor" will read the X-ray and review the results of the lab tests and make a home visit to see her. The nurse adds: "You will like the doctor."

In private, Jean shares with the nurse that her mother has been demanding and is wearing her down. Jean says her mother sleeps until noon, but stays up until dawn watching television, which she misinterprets because she can't hear it (e.g., Hannah thought the television said that local onions were poisoned and then she accused Jean of poisoning her). Jean describes efforts to be nice to her mother. She took her out to eat, but the next morning the mother did not recall going out to eat and accused Jean of starving her and holding her "prisoner in a dark place."

Hannah's son comes to visit, and in a moment of clarity she calls him by name and says, "Oh my, that woman in there must be your sister and she is trying to help me." Later Hannah refers again to Jean as "that woman" and does not seem to know her.

After reviewing the X-ray and lab tests, as well as the Mini Multi-State Examination and the past health history, and examining Hannah, the health care provider decides Hannah's hip is not broken and notes that she has a history of pernicious anemia and probably has Alzheimer's Disease. He writes orders for a B12 injection every week for three weeks, then every month; a home health aide for assistance with hygiene tasks; and prescribes 5 mg of donepezil (Aricept) daily.

Questions

1. Why did the nurse take time to chat with Hannah about her dog and fluff up her pillows? Why did the nurse check the batteries of the hearing aides and want her to wear hearing aides? What else does the nurse need to do at this point?

2. Why could the client identify her parents from an old picture and not recall the names of her children or grandchildren or the day, month, or year? Why can she recall words of songs, and what implications does this have for interventions?

3. Why did the nurse make a point of telling Hannah that the health care provider who would come would be very nice? What would you do or say differently if you were the nurse in this case? What in particular are the provider and nurse hoping to learn from the CBC, thyroid, and HIV laboratory tests?

4. The health care provider has diagnosed pernicious anemia for this client. Do you have reason to believe that pernicious anemia is the cause of this dementia? What is pernicious anemia?

5. What do you think of Jean's idea of taking the battery out of the car and letting Hannah try to start it every day?

6. If you were the nurse, would you mention to Hannah's daughter the possibility of having her mother declared incompetent in court at some point and becoming her mother's legal guardian?

7. The client's daughter asks you to explain what Alzheimer's Disease is. She also wants to know about the stages and incidence of Alzheimer's Disease. How would you respond to these questions?

8. What are the diagnostic criteria for dementia of the Alzheimer's type, and do you think this client matches those criteria?

9. Is there a definitive test for Alzheimer's Disease? What is the Mini Multi-State Exam that the health care provider ordered for Hannah?

10. What are the current theories of causation of Alzheimer's Disease?

11. What treatments are currently being used with Alzheimer's clients?

12. If you were the nurse in this case, what teaching would you do with the client and her daughter about donepezil (Aricept)? What do you need to know about the drug? If the client refuses to take her Aricept when offered by her daughter, what would you recommend?

13. The client's daughter says she has a fear and a reoccurring nightmare that she will eventually need to place her mother in a facility that cares for people with Alzheimer's, but she wants to keep her at home. Keeping in mind Black American culture, what questions, comments, or suggestions would you have for Jean at this time? Do you think Jean needs support, and if so, what kinds of support would you suggest?

14. What assessment data would you like to have if you were the nurse writing a nursing care plan for this client? What nursing diagnoses, goals, and interventions would you likely write for this client?

GENDER

Male

AGE

15

SETTING

- Alternative high school health classes with school nurse

ETHNICITY

- White American and Black American

CULTURAL CONSIDERATIONS

PREEXISTING CONDITIONS

- Learning disabilities

COEXISTING CONDITIONS

- Alcohol abuse

COMMUNICATION

DISABILITY

SOCIOECONOMIC

- Ward of state; qualifies for free school lunch

SPIRITUAL/RELIGIOUS

PHARMACOLOGIC

PSYCHOSOCIAL

- Current: sexually aggressive with girlfriend
- Early childhood: Father in prison
- Mother charged with neglect
- Multiple foster care situations

LEGAL

- On probation after serving sentence in juvenile justice system

ETHICAL

- Nurse contemplating adoption of client

ALTERNATIVE THERAPY

PRIORITIZATION

DELEGATION

CONDUCT DISORDER

Level of difficulty: High

Overview: Requires adhering to mental health principles that all people have worth and that all people can and do change. Requires maintaining a professional and helping therapeutic manner without losing sight of the need for setting consistent limits.

DIFFICULT

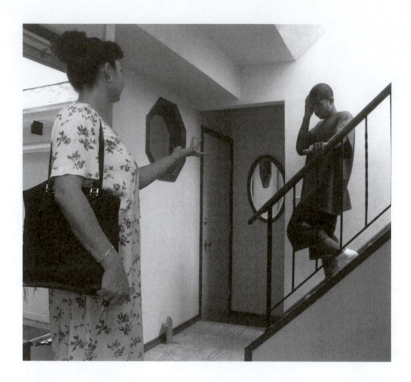

Client Profile

Elias is a 15-year-old male. His father is white American and his mother is black American. His father suddenly left the family when Elias was 7 years old. He later learned his father is in prison. Elias's mother tried to raise him and work two jobs. Elias started hanging out with a group of boys with a reputation for skipping school and drinking when he was 12 years old. A neighbor accused him of trying to drown her cat. He denied this, saying he was only trying to see if the cat could swim. The neighbor reported Elias's mother for neglect based on this and other instances of Elias getting into trouble while his mother was working. Elias became a ward of the state and was placed with a series of foster families. He has a reputation for starting fights and cutting a boy's face with his ring. The school expelled him because an ex-girlfriend accused him of threatening to hurt her if she didn't come back to him and have sex with him. The previous year a male student had killed his ex-girlfriend under similar circumstances, and the school was not about to risk a reoccurrence. In the past Elias has done some minor shoplifting without getting caught. About a year ago, he and some of his friends stole a car and decided to put on masks and costumes and rob people at knifepoint on Halloween. However, he chose an off-duty policeman to rob, and this ended in his being overpowered and arrested. He went to a state prison facility boot camp and a halfway house, then was placed with another foster family and returned to the public school system. He was not in the juvenile prison system long enough to get a GED and job training, but he did learn to live in a very structured system. Although he has learning disabilities, he made some progress in the prison education system in his reading skills.

Case Study

Elias is taking classes at an alternative high school with more flexible hours and programs for high school students who need to work, who have children, or who have been discipline problems and respond better in a structured, goal-oriented environment. Elias is taking a health course from a school nurse. The schools nurse gives Elias extra duties in the classroom and extra homework projects. He willingly completes the tasks. The school nurse tells Elias she is interested in his reading progress and offers to help him in reading or to assign a student with good reading skills to help him. The school nurse experienced trouble reading when she was a child, but received a lot of help and managed to compensate for some learning difficulties.

The school nurse receives a notice that she needs to come to a meeting of Elias's teachers and support staff. Elias has been having some discipline problems in one of his classes. The school nurse is surprised to hear this as Elias behaves well in health class.

In the faculty lounge waiting for the meeting about Elias to begin, the school nurse supervisor overhears two teachers talking about Elias. The general theme of their conversation is that they read his school records from the state juvenile corrections system and discovered that he has a diagnosis of Conduct Disorder (CD). One of the teachers says Elias is never going to amount to anything because he has Conduct Disorder. The other teacher says Elias is draining resources from other students as he will eventually go to prison. When the school nurse tries to talk with the teachers about Elias's good qualities, one of them suggests the school nurse adopt Elias if she likes him so well. The school nurse is not sure if the teacher is serious or not and begins to think the idea over.

Questions

1. If you were the school nurse in this case, would you have difficulty relating to Elias if he had been in prison for robbing someone at knifepoint? Would you treat him any differently if he had been imprisoned for doing or selling drugs? Describe an attitude and approach you and other nurses need to take with an adolescent like Elias.

2. Was the nurse's approach consisting of asking for assistance and offering to help with learning to read an acceptable approach or not? Provide a rationale for your answer. If you were the nurse in this case, how could you begin to work on developing empathy for Elias?

3. What criteria did Elias have to match to be diagnosed with Conduct Disorder? What behaviors does he have that match this diagnosis? Is it possible to have a mild case of Conduct Disorder, and what are the subtypes of Conduct Disorder?

4. Describe what keeps Elias from being diagnosed with Oppositional Defiant Disorder or Antisocial Personality Disorder instead of Conduct Disorder.

5. What are some theories about the cause of Conduct Disorder? What is the prevalence of Conduct Disorder?

6. What are learning disorders? Are learning disorders more common in adolescents with Conduct Disorder?

7. What data do you think would be most helpful to gather on this client? What nursing diagnoses and goals would you write for this client? What interventions would be helpful? Who do you need to work with in carrying out interventions?

8. What therapies are currently being used to treat Conduct Disorder? What is the likelihood that treatment of Conduct Disorder will have success?

9. Where would nurses encounter children and adolescents with diagnoses of Conduct Disorder other than the public school system?

10. Why is it important to care about and for children and adolescents who have a diagnosis of Conduct Disorder or who have traits of the diagnosis?

11. What do you think about the nurse's thought of adopting this client? What would you do in her place?

Martin

GENDER

Male

AGE

7

SETTING

- Community mental health center

ETHNICITY

- White American

CULTURAL CONSIDERATIONS

PREEXISTING CONDITION

COEXISTING CONDITION

COMMUNICATION

DISABILITY

SOCIOECONOMIC

SPIRITUAL/RELIGIOUS

PHARMACOLOGIC

- Methylphenidate hydrochloride (Concerta)

PSYCHOSOCIAL

LEGAL

ETHICAL

ALTERNATIVE THERAPY

PRIORITIZATION

DELEGATION

ATTENTION-DEFICIT/HYPERACTIVITY DISORDER

Level of difficulty: High

Overview: Requires the nurse to keep an open mind about whether a child with Attention-Deficit/ Hyperactivity Disorder (ADHD) might benefit from stimulant medication. Requires the nurse to discipline herself to neither advise for or against the medication, but to use the nursing process to assess an individual child's behavior, determine the child's problems (nursing diagnoses), and intervene in appropriate ways. Critical thinking is required to come up with creative ways to keep the child and others around him safe and to help him succeed in school when he has impulsivity, hyperactivity, and a short attention span.

Client Profile

Martin (Marty) is a 7-year-old boy who has a history of being so active that his family and others describe him like he is battery or motor-driven. He lives with his divorced father, two uncles, an aunt, and grandparents. His mother was given custody in divorce proceedings, but she changed her mind about caring for him as a single parent and left him with the father. Since that time Marty has only seen his mother once. The father intends to go to court for custody when he has money to pay the lawyer and court costs.

Marty has gone nonstop from the time he gets up until he goes to bed at night since he was a toddler. Marty seems to have no concern for safety. At age four he bit into a live lamp cord, resulting in a serious burn and scarring of his lip. This condition was corrected by plastic surgery. On a walk with a cousin, he suddenly climbed over the fence around an electrical transformer station and refused to get out. His attention span is short, and he goes from activity to activity quickly. One minute he is pointing a bow and arrow at a family member and the next jumping on the furniture. When he was four years old, he discovered the fun of doing somersaults in the tub, and those supervising him fear he is going to hit his head on the faucets. The family takes turns watching him as he quickly tires a person out. Family members have noticed when they send him to get something he forgets to bring it back.

His teacher at school has sent notes home and had conferences to communicate his behavior at school, including interrupting others, not wanting to wait his turn, and not following directions like other children. His hand is frequently up, and he has something to say whether it is relevant or not. When other children are finishing work, he is doing something else. He gets out of his seat frequently. When the teacher gets him to sit in his seat and do his work, she notices his hands and feet are very "fidgety" and he makes careless mistakes. He seldom turns in assigned homework. His grandparents try to get him to read for them, but he says: "I don't want to." They find it nearly impossible to get him to sit and play quietly. The family and the teacher have all noticed that he is easily distracted by anything happening in his environment. He is an attractive child with a handsome smile. People tend to like him even though they don't like some of his behavior.

Case Study

Marty and his father have come to the community mental health center. Several people have suggested to the father that Marty might have ADHD. If he has this disorder, the father wants to see if the child psychiatrist will prescribe some medication and/or offer other help to increase Marty's attention span and slow him down a bit. Marty is into everything in the waiting room. He takes things out of the trash receptacle, throws some toys at the desk, climbs over and under chairs, turns the lights off and on, and then he runs behinds the desk and grabs one of the donuts the nursing staff have for coffee break. The father says to the nurse: "I'm sorry. Do you think he has ADHD?"

The nurse weighs Marty, measures his height, and gets vital signs and a preliminary history. The psychologist does some testing and asks a lot of questions and verifies the diagnosis of ADHD. The child psychiatrist also sees Marty and his father and prescribes methylphenidate hydrochloride (Concerta). The nurse does some teaching with the father and answers his questions. Next, the nurse asks the father about Marty's mother. The father reveals that the mother has custody of the child, but that the child lives with him. The nurse gets a release of information from the father so the treatment team can share information and obtain information from the mother. The nurse contracts the mother in regard to the medication. The mother says, "I don't want Marty to have Ritalin or any other drug that messes with his mind. I won't sign giving permission for him to be on drugs." She says: "I have read that Ritalin is prescribed for kids that don't need it. Marty just has more energy than most kids his age. He will grow out of it."

Questions

1. If you were the nurse in this case, what would you say to the father when he asks: "Do you think he (Marty) has ADHD?"

2. If you were the nurse in this case, what could you and other staff members do to make the time in the waiting room easier for the father and this very active child?

3. What behaviors does Marty have that match the criteria for Attention-Deficit/Hyperactivity Disorder (ADHD)? Looking at the criteria, what type of ADHD do you think he would most likely have?

4. What would you tell the father about Concerta, the medication prescribed for his son?

5. If you had the opportunity, what would you say to the mother who is refusing to allow Ritalin for Marty and stating he just has more energy than other boys and will grow out of his hyperactivity?

6. Discuss the debate as to whether ADHD is overdiagnosed and Ritalin and similar stimulants are overprescribed for ADHD. Is Ritalin or other psychostimulants sometimes necessary for children? Why or why not?

7. What other medications besides Ritalin could the health care provider prescribe for ADHD?

8. The father asks: What causes ADHD? How would you answer this question?

9. Marty's father shares an observation that all the children he knows that have ADHD seem to be boys. He asks: "Do girls also have ADHD? What is the ratio of girls to boys who have ADHD?" How would you answer this father?

10. If you were to help write a care plan for this client, what information would you like to gather?

11. What nursing diagnoses and goals would you likely write for this client? What interventions, other than medication, do you think would be helpful for this client?

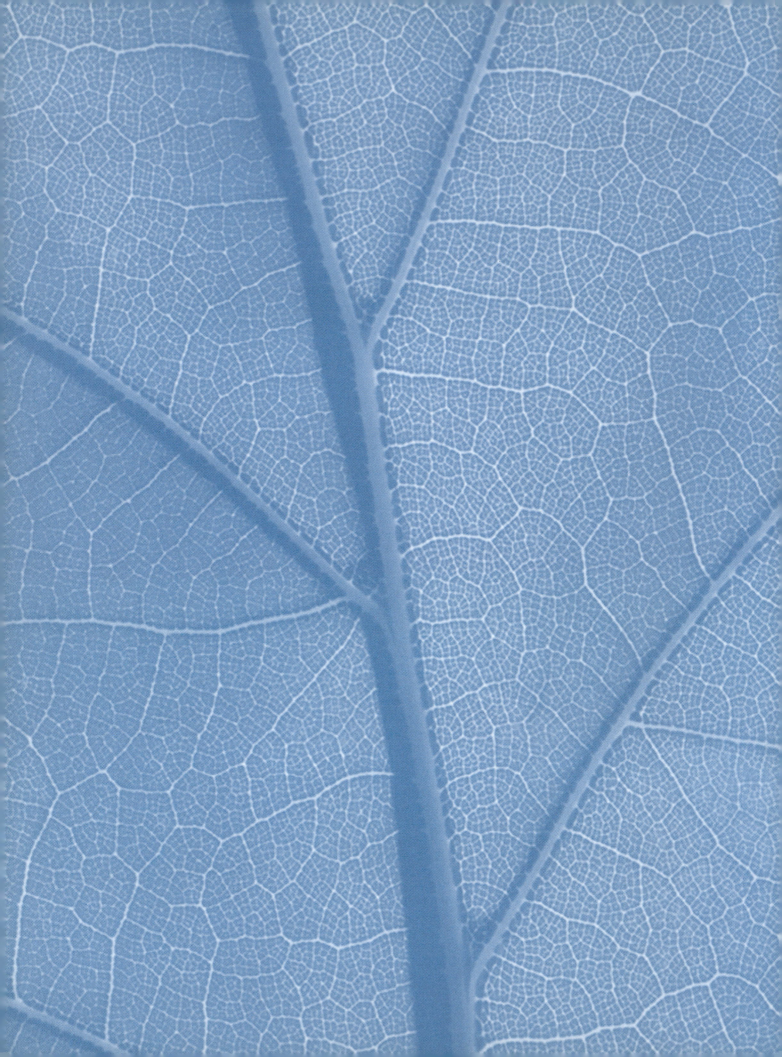

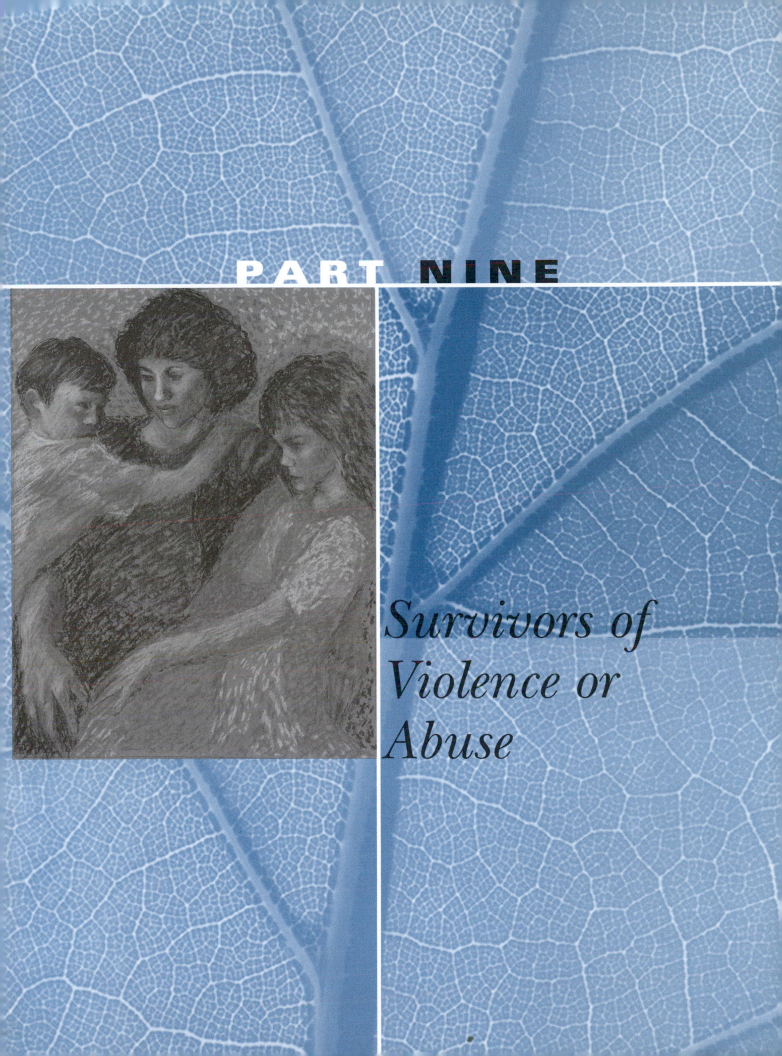

PART NINE

Survivors of Violence or Abuse

Reata

GENDER

Female

AGE

10

SETTING

- Home setting with visit by home health nurse

ETHNICITY

- White American

CULTURAL CONSIDERATIONS

- Southern
- Rural
- Military

PREEXISTING CONDITIONS

COEXISTING CONDITIONS

COMMUNICATION

DISABILITY

SOCIOECONOMIC

- Lower middle class

SPIRITUAL/RELIGIOUS

- Belongs to Seventh-Day Adventist church but not attending

PHARMACOLOGIC

PSYCHOSOCIAL

LEGAL

- Legal requirement to report "suspected" abuse
- Confidentiality

ETHICAL

- Child and mother's need to report suspected child abuse to ensure safety.

ALTERNATIVE THERAPY

PRIORITIZATION

DELEGATION

PHYSICAL ABUSE OF A CHILD

Level of difficulty: Moderate

Overview: Requires understanding of what constitutes child abuse and critical thinking to determine if there is sufficient evidence to warrant a suspicion of abuse. Requires knowledge of the legal requirements and process for reporting child abuse.

Client Profile

Reata is a 10-year-old girl living with her parents in their rural home. Her mother suffers from Manic Depression and Panic Disorder with Agoraphobia and smokes two packages of cigarettes a day. When agitated or angry, the mother hits Reata or burns her with cigarettes and tells her that she was/is an unwanted child. Reata's mother was raised in the Seventh-Day Adventist Church by the grandparents who live in a nearby city and still attend church. Reata's mother does not attend due to her Agoraphobia and her mental illness, which, combined with living in a rural area, greatly isolates the family.

Reata's father is a member of a military guard unit and is gone from home for long periods of time. When the father is home, he punishes Reata for such things as not doing chores perfectly, not having better grades, imperfect table manners, and for many small infractions of his strict rules. She is beaten with his belt and sent to her room hungry. One time she tried to run away, but her father killed her dog and put his head on the fence for her to see when he found her and brought her back home. She is afraid of her father and more so of his belt.

During the time that the father is gone, Reata tries to stay away from home as much as possible and to hide from her mother when she is at home. She feels safer when the visiting nurse is in the home and comes out of hiding due to curiosity and in hopes of getting some food or candy without being beaten or burned.

Case Study

The visiting nurse knocks on the door, which is opened by Reata, who is wearing a cast on her arm. The nurse is a visiting nurse from the county health department who has come to care for Reata's mother. The nurse asks Reata: "How are you today?" The child whispers in a low voice: "Hungry." The mother yells: "I heard that. It is not mealtime yet. Go get the nurse and me a glass of ice water, you stupid girl." The mother tells the nurse: "She just wants to eat all the time. I can't fill her up no matter how hard I try."

The nurse says: "Reata seems very thin." The mother does not respond, and the nurse asks how much Reata weighs. The mother responds: "Oh, I don't know how much she weighs, but the worthless child eats all the time and just runs it all off. She is always running. Don't worry about her. Take my blood pressure." The nurse starts getting out her stethoscope and sphygmomanometer. She quietly slips Reata a sandwich from her bag while the mother is walking toward her chair and not looking. The nurse can see Reata in the next room, sitting under the table and eating the sandwich in a few quick bites, without her mother being aware of it.

Midway through the visit, the nurse says: "I notice that Reata has a cast on." The mother does not reply, and the nurse says: "Tell me about the cast." The mother explains: "She is a clumsy girl. Always climbing trees and falling out. She also climbs out her window and jumps off the roof [one-story roof]." The nurse notices a burn on the dorsal side of Reata's left hand, but says nothing about it at this time, focusing instead on the client, Reata's mother. Just before leaving, the nurse says: "Reata has a burn on her hand." "Just a cooking accident because she is stupid," replies the mother.

Questions

1. If you were the nurse in this case, making a first visit and not knowing what was going on in the family, what would you think when you see Reata's cast and her thinness and hear her say she is hungry? What would you think as you hear the mother's explanations for these observations and for the burn on the child's hand?

2. If you were the nurse, would your visit focus only on the mother's care or would you be concerned with her child? Did the nurse do the right thing in giving the child a sandwich, and what did the nurse learn by doing this?

3. Briefly describe the therapeutic communication tools used by the nurse in this home visit and a rationale for using them. What strategy does the nurse use to get information about the daughter from the client? Do you agree with this strategy, and if so, why? If not, what strategy would you like to use?

4. If you were the nurse in this case, what would you do to build a trusting relationship with Reata and help her other than reporting your suspicion of abuse? Provide a rationale for your actions.

5. Discuss the federal act that names and defines four major classifications of maltreatment of children. As the nurse in this case, your observations and assessment in the home would best support a suspicion of which one or more of the four types of abuse described in the federal act?

6. What are some of the common characteristics of parents who abuse or neglect children? Do Reata's parents or family have any of these characteristics?

7. What are some behaviors frequently found in children who are abused? What conditions could a child have that might mislead a nurse into thinking the child was being abused when they are not experiencing abuse?

8. What short-term and long-term effects could occur if this child is being abused and neglected and this continues because you don't report your suspicions to the proper authorities?

9. Are all nurses legally obligated to report suspected child abuse? Does the nurse have to gather sufficient data to prove child abuse? Are you as a nurse protected from civil and criminal liability if, acting in the interest of a child, you report suspected child abuse or neglect? How can you find out the procedure to follow to report child abuse and neglect?

10. What do you think bothers nurses the most about reporting suspicion of abuse and neglect? If you report that you suspect Reata is being abused and neglected and she is taken from the family and placed in foster care, how would you feel? On the other hand, if you report suspected abuse and neglect and the authorities decide your suspicions are unwarranted or that the child is in no danger and better off staying with her parents, how would you feel and what would you do?

11. What other means of getting information can you think of to confirm your suspicion of physical abuse and neglect, or to rule it out?

12. Making the child as well as the mother, who is the official client of the nurse, the focus of nursing process, what additional assessments would you do? What nursing diagnoses and goals would you likely write for this child if you continue working with the family and child? What interventions would be helpful?

CASE STUDY 2

Francis

GENDER

Male

AGE

77

SETTING

- Gerontologist's office

ETHNICITY

- White American

CULTURAL CONSIDERATIONS

PREEXISTING CONDITION

COEXISTING CONDITION

COMMUNICATION

- Hard of hearing; has hearing aides

DISABILITY

SOCIOECONOMIC

- Middle income

SPIRITUAL/RELIGIOUS

PHARMACOLOGIC

- haloperidol (Haldol)

PSYCHOSOCIAL

- Daughter controls access of client to others

LEGAL

- Legal requirement in most, if not all, states for nurses to report abuse/neglect of elderly
- Confidentiality
- Right to make decisions unless declared incompetent

ETHICAL

- Professional manner with a person suspected of abusing the elderly
- Daughter giving client medication without his consent

PRIORITIZATION

DELEGATION

PHYSICAL ABUSE OF ELDERLY CLIENT

Level of difficulty: High

Overview: Requires knowledge of signs and symptoms of elder abuse. Requires keeping an open mind while using therapeutic communication skills to determine if there is enough evidence to warrant reporting suspected elder abuse.

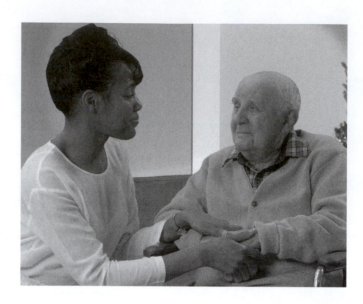

Client Profile

Francis, described as a cantankerous old man by family and neighbors, lived alone until recently, when he reluctantly moved to another city to live with his daughter Alline. He has five living children, none of whom particularly like him, remembering him as being humorless and even mean to them when they were growing up. Francis feared going to a nursing home and got his daughter Alline to promise to keep him out of nursing homes by saying he would leave her some money when he dies.

Alline thought it was a good idea to have her father move in with her, but it soon became evident that he required a lot of care, could not be left alone safely, and was never quite satisfied with anything she did for him. Alline also had to care for his dog that he brought with him, and she did not like the dog. Alline began to resent her siblings not helping her with their father's care. One day she became so angry with her father, the dog, her siblings, and the situation that she shoved her father. He fell, broke his glasses, broke a bone in his foot, and acquired a few bruises. There was some question about whether the foot was broken or not, but Alline decided it probably was not broken. She thought it would be a lot of trouble to get the foot x-rayed, so she did not. A few days later Alline lost control again and hit her father several times, giving him even more bruises. Francis has hearing aids, but his daughter has not put batteries in them. He is usually restrained in a wheel-chair when his daughter goes to the store to get groceries. Francis often feels like he is drugged and wonders if his daughter is slipping something into his pudding to calm him down. He usually slips the dog at least half his pudding. Francis is correct in his suspicions. Alline's neighbor gave her a bottle of Haldol after her husband died and no longer needed it. Alline has been putting half a crushed Haldol pill into the pudding.

Case Study

Francis's daughter and a younger brother, who came from another state on an unannounced visit, bring Francis to a gerontologist's office. The brother tells the nurse that he is concerned about Francis's swollen foot, his complaint of pain, the bruising, and Francis thinking it had been at least three years since he had last seen a doctor. The brother mentions that Francis cannot see well because his glasses were broken and he does not hear well because his hearing aids don't work. After weighing Francis, the nurse tells the family she is taking him to an examination room for his physical examination. Alline jumps up to go with them. Francis yells, "No, don't come!" Alline insists on accompanying her father and says: "The nurse will have trouble understanding you and you will have trouble understanding and remembering, so I had better come too."

Questions

1. What are some possible reasons this elderly client might not want his daughter with him during his physical examination?

2. The client is hard of hearing. What actions will you take to enhance his ability to hear you?

3. What approach will you take with this client whom you suspect might be the victim of elder abuse? Are there questions that need to be asked of the caregiver and the client separately? If so, what are these questions and what is your rationale for interviewing the client and others separately?

4. Define elder abuse, elder physical abuse, and elder neglect. Give examples of caretaker behavior that constitutes elder physical abuse and elder neglect. What is the incidence of elder abuse? Are more men than women victims of elder abuse?

5. What are the risk factors for elder abuse? Which of these risk factors are present in this case? What are the signs and symptoms of elder physical abuse that you would look for? What are the signs and symptoms of neglect you would be observing for?

6. If this client says nothing to you (the nurse) or to the health care provider about abuse and he is being abused, why isn't he telling you about the abuse and getting it stopped? Are you as a nurse required to report suspected elder abuse, and how do you report it?

7. If you report suspected elder abuse and it is substantiated, can the abuser be punished by the legal system? What percentage of reported suspected elder abuse cases are substantiated, and what is the type of elder abuse most often substantiated?

8. If the client and his daughter hold firm in that nothing abusive is occurring in the household, what is your course of action?

9. The client says he thinks his daughter is putting pills in his pudding. Alline admits to getting the deceased neighbor's Haldol (haloperidol) and putting it into her father's food. What actions do you need to take? Given what you know and suspect about how Alline is treating her father, how would you now feel about working with Alline and her father?

10. Nurses in some health care providers' offices may not write care plans; however, some likely nursing diagnoses will come to your mind. What are those nursing diagnoses? What goals and interventions would be helpful to this client?

11. What do you especially need to document in this and other cases of suspected abuse?

GENDER

Male

AGE

11

SETTING

- Deaf school infirmary

ETHNICITY

- Mother is White American; father is Hispanic American

CULTURAL CONSIDERATIONS

- Hispanic

PREEXISTING CONDITION

- Waardenburg Syndrome (WS)
- Possible Hirschsprung Disease associated with WS

COEXISTING CONDITION

- Urine infection with low grade fever

COMMUNICATION

- Congenital deafness; uses American Sign Language

DISABILITY

- Congenital deafness

SOCIOECONOMIC

- Upper middle class

SPIRITUAL/RELIGIOUS

- Catholic

PHARMACOLOGIC

PSYCHOSOCIAL

LEGAL

- Legal requirements to report suspected child abuse

ETHICAL

- Unethical to ask questions out of curiosity rather than need to know

ALTERNATIVE THERAPY

PRIORITIZATION

DELEGATION

SEXUAL ABUSE OF A CHILD

Level of difficulty: High

Overview: Requires critical thinking, as well as knowledge of the laws pertaining to reporting of suspected sexual abuse of a child, to determine a course of action to take when a deaf child describes experiences that suggest sexual abuse by his father. Requires knowledge of the communication needs of deaf children and critical thinking to determine how to meet those needs.

DIFFICULT

Client Profile

Chuy, an 11-year-old boy, was born deaf in both ears. At first both eyes looked the same color, but after awhile it was very noticeable that one eye was bright blue and the other brown. His father, a third-generation Hispanic American, blamed the mother for this problem, saying she had bad genes. The paternal grandfather blamed his estranged sister for putting the evil eye on the boy. The neonatologist and the otologist blamed it on Waardenburg Syndrome (WS); their assessments found the father carries the trait, and several members of his family, including the boy's grandfather, have a variety of signs associated with WS, but none are deaf like Chuy.

The father physically and emotionally abused the mother. He was angry with her for producing an imperfect child and angry at the child for not being perfect. The father began to sexually abuse Chuy at about age 4. When the boy went to a residential school for the deaf, the mother went to work, separated from the father, and eventually divorced him. The court decision was joint custody. The mother knew of the sexual abuse, but did not report it or use it in the divorce trial.

Case Study

Chuy is admitted to the school infirmary for observation because he complains of a stomachache and he has a low grade fever. He is found to have urine infection. The infirmary nurse has two other children under her care, and they are isolated with chicken pox. The nurse is able to assess Chuy in a private area of the infirmary. She first plays a game of "Go Fish" and gets him to take turns with her telling "silly jokes." She then takes his vital signs and listens to his heart and lungs and lets him listen to his own heartbeat. The nurse listens for bowel sounds and palpates the stomach, inquiring about pain and about when he had last "pooped." Chuy says maybe three days ago when he was home with his father, but since coming back to school, he is having a hard time pooping. "So it was easier to 'poop' at home," the nurse says. Chuy reveals that his father puts his finger up his "butt" and puts other objects up there to stretch the "butt" and help the "poop" come out. "So he helps you …" the nurse says, and Chuy responds: "He helps other people too by taking pictures of how he does this so they will learn to do it, and he sometimes lets them practice on me or do other things with my wee wee and takes pictures. Oh, I am not supposed to tell. My dad told me to keep it secret. He said other people won't understand and they will be jealous. I won't be punished for telling will I, nurse? Dad says I will be punished if I tell and my mom will get real sick and die if I tell. Please don't tell anyone."

Questions

1. Describe Waardenburg Syndrome (WS), including signs and symptoms.

2. What possible reason or reasons did the nurse in this case have for beginning an assessment by first playing "Go Fish" and taking turns telling silly jokes with this client?

3. What do you suppose could be the cause of this child's constipation? What assessments could you do if you were the nurse in this case?

4. What do you think the nurse in this case might think or feel as the child describes his father's behavior associated with his (the client's) genitals? What techniques did the nurse in the case study use in examining the client and why?

5. How would you define sexual abuse of a child? Are there some gray areas about what is sexual abuse and what is not sexual abuse?

Questions (continued)

6. Do you need to ask this client questions about the sexual abuse to make sure the child was sexually abused and to get more specific details of the abuse (i.e., take a sexual abuse history)? If yes, what is your rationale? If no, should someone else do this, and if so, who and why?

7. What do you need to do and say in response to the child's request that you tell no one about the things his father did to him? What thoughts do you have about documentation of the child's statements in regard to his treatment by his father? Should you take notes while the child is talking?

8. What reasons could the mother have for not reporting the sexual abuse of her son? Should you ask her? Do you need to know the reasons?

9. If this client is to have an anogenital examination, what preparation would be helpful to the child? What is usually done in an anogenital examination? What would it mean if the anogenital examination were negative for evidence of sexual abuse?

10. What behavioral symptoms do sexually abused children display? Will all children who have been sexually abused display behavioral symptoms? What are some thoughts and feelings children have identified in regard to their sexual abuse?

11. What is the incidence of sexual abuse of children? Do you think the incidence is similar or different in other countries? Do you think culture plays any role in this case?

12. Are sexual abuse rates the same for boys as for girls? Do you think that sexual abuse rates are higher for disabled children? If yes, why do you think this is so?

13. When children are sexually abused, who is often the perpetrator? Is this the same for other forms of abuse?

14. What nursing diagnoses and goals would you likely write for this client? What interventions do you think would be helpful for this client?

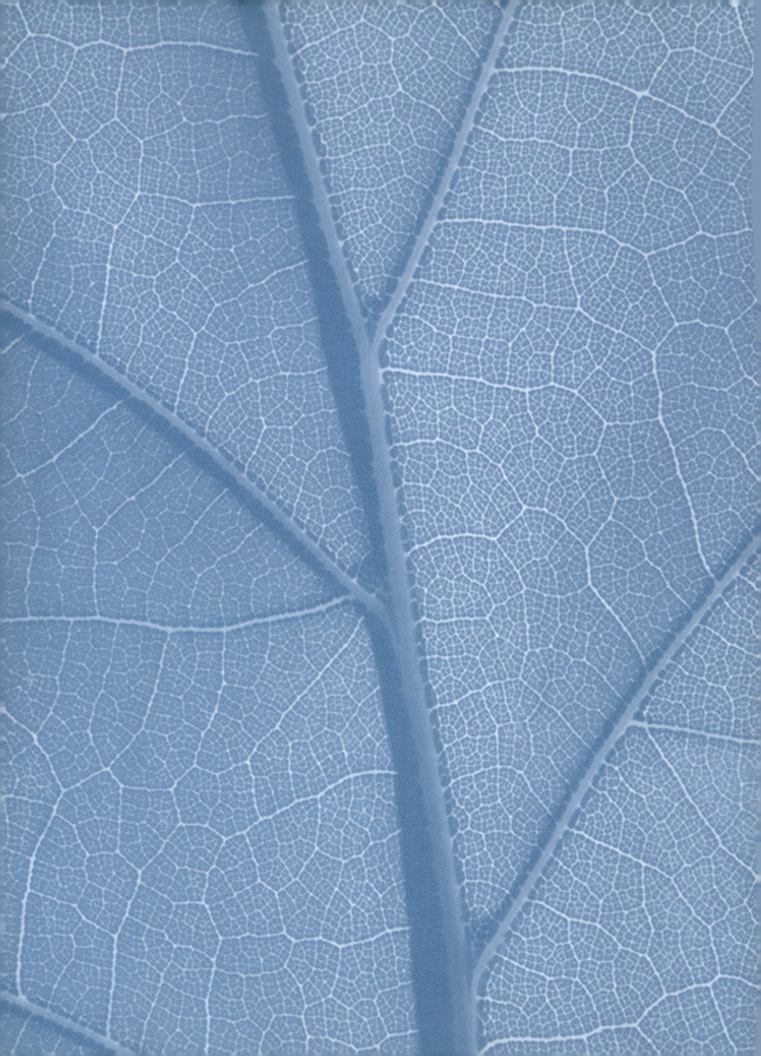

Index